HOME GYM FITNESS
EXERCISE BIKE
WORKOUTS

DR. CHARLES T. KUNTZLEMAN

CONTEMPORARY
BOOKS, INC.
CHICAGO

Library of Congress Cataloging in Publication Data

Kuntzleman, Charles T.
    Exercise bike workouts.

    (Home gym fitness)
    1. Exercise—Equipment and supplies. 2. Bicycles.

I. Title.   II. Series: Kuntzleman, Charles T.
Home gym fitness
GV543.K86   1985   613.7′028   85-5775
ISBN 0-8092-5271-6

Table on page 115 reprinted with permission by *Runner's World* Magazine Company, Inc., 1400 Stierlin Road, Mountain View, California 94043.

Published by Contemporary Books, Inc.
180 North Michigan Avenue, Chicago, Illinois 60601
Manufactured in the United States of America
International Standard Book Number: 0-8092-5271-6

Published simultaneously in Canada by Beaverbooks, Ltd.
195 Allstate Parkway, Valleywood Business Park
Markham, Ontario L3R 4T8 Canada

CONTENTS

ACKNOWLEDGMENTS

THE FOLLOWING COMPANIES supplied equipment and clothing for the photographs in *Home Gym Fitness: Exercise Bike Workouts*.

BICYCLING EQUIPMENT

BodyGuard 990
J. Oglaend, Inc.
40 Radio Circle, Mt. Kisco, NY 10549-0096

Fitness Products
Box 254, Hillsdale, MI 49242

Monark Bicycle
Universal Fitness Products
50 Commercial St., Plainview, L.I., NY 11803

Schwinn XR-8 and Schwinn Air-Dyne
Excelsior Fitness Equipment Co.
615 Landwehr Rd., Northbrook, IL 60062

WEIGHT-TRAINING EQUIPMENT

Universal Weights
Universal
PO Box 1270, Cedar Rapids, IA 52406

BICYCLING CLOTHING

Men's Biking Shorts and Shirt
Women's Biking Shorts and Shirt
Bell Wether
1161 Mission St., San Francisco, CA 94103

Men's and Women's Biking Gloves
Men's and Women's Biking Shoes
Men's and Women's Biking Socks
Cannondale Corp.
Friendship Rd., RD #6, Bedford, PA 15522

PREFACE

THE $16 BILLION sporting goods industry is undergoing a revolution: home fitness sales are skyrocketing. Home exercise sales have doubled in the past two years, and 31 million Americans now claim they have exercise equipment at home. In 1984 $1 billion was spent by people like you on home fitness equipment.

While it is true that much of the home gym and exercise equipment is purchased by higher-income consumers, it is equally true that economy-minded consumers have found it less expensive to use exercise equipment at home than to purchase a health club membership.

People today are interested in self-improvement. They are looking for ways to relieve stress and remain active. The upwardly mobile group is becoming more affluent and able to afford quality equipment.

The most popular home equipment items purchased today are exercise bicycles, jogging trampolines, multi-gyms, free weights, and rowing machines. A 1984 survey of home fitness products indicated that sales of stationary bicycles jumped nearly 70 percent over the last two years, going from 1.5 million units to nearly 2.5 million units. In addition, Americans bought 3 million sets of barbells, almost 500,000 rowing machines, 1.5 million jogging trampolines, and 750,000 multipurpose gyms.

The interest in health and fitness is expected to continue at least through 1990. A recent Gallup poll showed that 59 percent of all adults exercise daily. That is 12 percent more than in 1982 and double the 1961 figure.

This book is one in a series for Contemporary Books that tells you, the consumer, how to get the most out of your recently purchased equipment. The series, titled *Home Gym Fitness*, includes three books focusing on three of the most popular pieces of equipment—stationary bicycles, rowing machines, and free weights.

Diversified Products (DP) sells 15 percent of all home exercise equipment. The next-largest companies are Huffy, AMF-Whitely, AMEREC, and Vitamaster. While these are dominant forces in the marketplace today, there are plenty of other smaller suppliers and manufacturers. Thomas B. Doyle, director of information and research for the National Sporting Goods Association, estimated in 1984 that there are 150 manufacturers fighting for a piece of the home exercise market.

Because of the "hotness" of the market, some heavy hitters are also entering the field. The Campbell Soup Company, for example, has recently acquired the Triangle Manufacturing Company of Raleigh, North Carolina—a company that manufactures dumbbells. West Bend, a division of Dart Industries, bought out Total Gym in July 1983 and in April 1984 purchased PreCor—a manufacturer of treadmills, rowing machines, and exercise bicycles.

Historically, most of the home fitness sales have been made through chain stores—Sears, J. C. Penney, K-Mart, and Montgomery Ward. While sales are still strong in the chain stores, many people now purchase from their favorite sporting goods dealer or from a new phenomenon—a sales representative who makes house calls. Regardless of where and how you purchase your equipment, these salespeople are valuable resources. They, along with the contents of this book, will show you how to get the most out of your home fitness equipment.

Home Gym Fitness: Exercise Bike Workouts discusses various types of stationary bicycles and cycle ergometers. So read and enjoy *Home Gym Fitness: Exercise Bike Workouts*. It will help you maximize the use of your exercise bike and reach new levels of fitness and exercise enjoyment.

1

THE BASICS

YOU'RE PROBABLY LIKE many Americans—you're exercising at home. Costly and crowded health clubs have driven you to the point where you are searching for creative and cost-effective ways to work out at home. Also like many Americans, you've decided that the exercise bicycle is best.

According to *The New York Times*, Americans bought almost 2.5 million exercise bicycles in 1983—worth $275 million, retail. In 1981 a modest 1.5 million units were sold. Industry analysts say that 1984 was a banner year. While all the information is not in, it appears that at least 3 million units were sold. The latter figure may be the subject of industry hype, but one thing is clear: the exercise bicycle is one of the most popular pieces of indoor exercise equipment.

Another thing is clear: the quality of construction, and hence the durability, of the home exercise bike is rapidly improving. In the 1960s, with the exception of Schwinn indoor bicycles and one or two produced by other relatively unknown manufacturers, most home exercise bikes were pieces of junk. Poor construction, fragile components, and few options made these bikes dangerous to ride, difficult to sit on, and undependable. Indoor bikes had a bad reputation—nice to look at, but rarely used.

In America's basements and attics today you'll find exercise bikes of the '60s collecting dust and rust or going for $10 (or less) at neighborhood garage sales. No one wants these $39.95 specials. They shake, wobble, pinch the skin, provide an uneven pedaling movement, and are noisy beyond belief. Why, you can't even watch TV without the volume blaring above the noise of the bicycle. I had one. The bike lasted 15 riding hours before the handlebars and seat wiggled loose and the pedaling action became uneven and distracting.

Fortunately, high technology has pushed the exercise bicycle toward the 21st century. Many companies have responded to the demand of the market for quality equipment that will last for years and, with proper care, maybe a lifetime. Exercise bicycles help the exerciser condition the heart and lungs, provide a good means of expending calories, and firm the legs. They're durable, quiet, and have options that can make indoor bicycling fun.

Today, it's a buyer's market when it comes to exercise bicycling. At least 20 companies supply a great variety of exercise bicycles. The number of companies is bound to increase as entrepreneurs and big companies see opportunities in an industry that is just starting to emerge.

The products offered to consumers are diverse. Some retail for $59.95; others have been priced as high as $3,995. The latter bike has an impressive array of mind-boggling electronic gadgetry that is largely unnecessary, unless you are buying a gift for the person who has everything.

Don't let the $3,995 price tag scare you, though. A quality indoor bike can be purchased for slightly more than $200. In fact, most of the quality exercise bikes range between $250 and $600.

While you probably have already purchased your bike, it is clear that if you spent more than $300 you bought bells and whistles and other paraphernalia that are nice but not necessary. A basic $250 bike will help you firm your calves, buttocks, and thighs just as well as the $1,995 model. The $250 bike will allow you to condition your heart and lungs and burn calories just as efficiently as the $3,995 electronic wizard. The extra hundreds of dollars will not make you any more fit, although the gadgetry will make your indoor cycling more interesting and fun. The difference is similar to the difference between going on a trip in a Chevy and in a BMW.

But before we go too far down the road, a distinction between exercise bicycles is necessary. Currently, there are two basic kinds of products on the market—exercise bicycles and cycle ergometers. There are some hybrids, but the key is to understand the differences between an exercise bike and an ergometer.

A BICYCLE OR AN ERGOMETER?

To the average person on the street, a bicycle you ride indoors is a stationary bike or an exercise bike, regardless of the gadgets attached. To the scientist, however, there are substantial differences.

In their simplest form, both a bicycle and an ergometer will help you condition your body. The difference is that, with an ordinary exercise bike, you can *feel* your condition getting better. An ergometer will *tell* you, in figures, how much better.

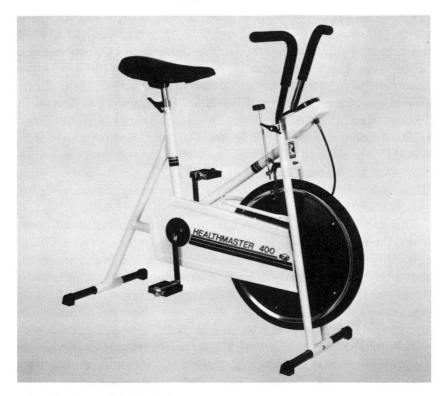

The Roadmaster Healthmaster 400

The home exercise bicycle is available in a wide range of models and prices. Stationary exercise bicycles are exactly what their name implies—bicycles that remain stationary as you pedal. They come in all shapes and sizes. They look like any other bicycle except one wheel is missing. Usually, exercise bicycles are made of 1-inch to 1½-inch welded tubular steel. There are extrawide front and rear legs and dual rear stabilizer struts for stability. The handlebars are usually made of chrome. The pedals turn a sprocket and chain to drive the wheel.

The frame of the bike usually has a variable resistance device that allows you to increase or decrease pedal pressure or resistance to pedaling. While resistance devices make your pedaling more difficult (or easier), the exercise bikes are not calibrated. So you have no way of knowing how much work you are doing. You can "feel" that you are working harder or easier. You can even check your heart rate to verify it. But you won't know *exactly* how much work you are doing. So, when you get on a different bicycle, you have no idea of what resistance to set on the dial. You must guess, feel, or estimate the amount of work you are doing. Even if the resistance dial has numbers on it, there is no assurance that a "5" on Bike A is the same as "5" on Bike B.

Some of the exercise bicycle brand names are Bianchi Exerciser, Bodyguard 955 Home/Club Bike, Bodyguard 957 Triathlon Trainer Racing Bike, DP 2000, DP Body Shaper, Fitness 1000, Huffy Aerobic Fitness Cycle, Jayfro Fleetline, Monark 877 Professional Exercise Cycle, Rabbit Home Cycle, Rowen Exercise Cycle, Schwinn XR-8, Swedish Flywheel Bike, Tunturi Home Cycle, Vitamaster Dual Action Exerciser, Vitamaster Slender Cycle, and Walton Carousel Jogger.

The cycle ergometer is similar to, yet substantially different from, the exercise bike. Most ergometers look like exercise bicycles. They have handlebars, pedals, bike seat, chain and sprocket, one wheel, and a sturdy frame. A speedometer, odometer, and timer are also present. There are surface differences as well. Cycle ergometers appear to be better built, have heavier components, and have more dials than exercise bicycles.

The real difference between the cycle ergometers and the exercise bicycles is that the ergometers allow you to set the exact pedaling resistance and compare that to internationally recognized work units. On ergometers, you can specifically calculate the work accomplished.

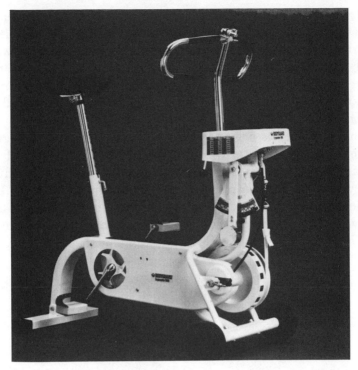

The Bodyguard 990 Ergometer   Photo courtesy of Bodyguard

Obviously, physicians and researchers like this feature. A physician can test a patient in the office and then provide specific recommendations to be followed at home. That makes the exercise safe and precise—a true exercise prescription. Likewise, a coach or an exercise physiologist can design a specific program for an athlete based on his or her own individual physical working capacity. Therefore, the conditioning program is tailor-made for the athlete, and the coach has the confidence that the work load is appropriate.

Surprisingly, many indoor exercisers who own cycle ergometers treat their ergometers as exercise bikes. They do not take advantage of the ergometer's features. That is OK, but that approach does not allow the exerciser to get his or her money's worth from the ergometer. How to do that is discussed in Chapter 5.

At first, the additional features of the cycle ergometer may not seem important to you, but if you really get serious about cycle fitness, you'll find the added features of the ergometer interesting, challenging, and a real asset to your training.

Ergometers may be mechanical or electronic. Mechanical ergometers for home use have been around since the early 1950s. Electronic ergometers appeared in the late 1960s, but it wasn't until the 1980s that they made a dent in the market. Priced between $2,000 and $4,000, electronic ergometers have a limited market, but their popularity is increasing rapidly, especially in health clubs.

Some of the cycle ergometer brand names include Bodyguard Ergometer 990, Cybex Fitron, Monark Mark II—Model 865, Monark 868 Testing Ergometer, Schwinn AirDyne, Schwinn BioDyne 2, Tunturi Ergometer, and Vitamaster Pro-1000. Electronic ergometers include Amerec EL-400, Bally Lifecycle 5000, Biocycle, Tunturi Electronic Ergometer, Universal Aerobicycle, and Wimbleton Industries Heart Mate.

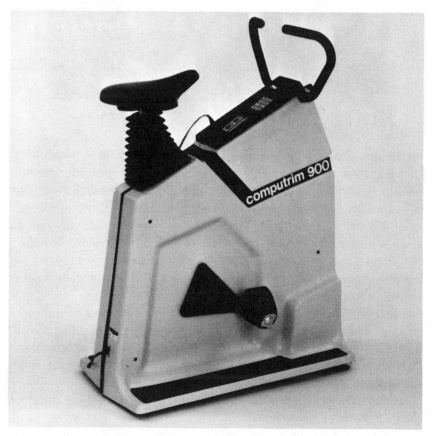

An electronic ergometer

ROLLERS AND WIND TRAINERS

Recently, outdoor cyclists have turned to a third type of device for indoor cycling—rollers and wind trainers. While these devices are rarely used or purchased by fitness buffs and remain the domain of outdoor cyclists, they are discussed here to make you aware of their availability and purpose.

The bicycle rollers and/or wind-load trainers allow you to ride your own bike indoors. The rollers are nothing more than that. They have three drums positioned so that you can mount your bike on the rollers and simulate riding outdoors (see photos on pages 6 and 7). While it's true that these devices don't have the same resistance as road riding, and getting off and on rollers can be awkward, rollers do help you develop pedal action, balance, leg speed, and cardiovascular fitness. But since resistance is minimal, development of leg strength is quite low.

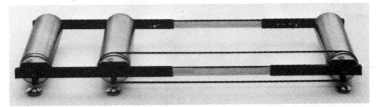

The Cinelli Home Trainer

Jeff Spencer, former California State Champion cyclist, says that riding rollers is difficult at first, but there are some tips that can help. At first, you have to find an appropriate speed. Riding either too fast or too slowly can be hazardous. Too much speed can cause the wheels to start hopping until you lose control of the bike. Riding too slowly creates control problems. He suggests that about 80 rpm in an intermediate gear works well. Next, you should not ride no-handed or standing up. Third, concentration is important. If you let your mind wander as you may at times in outdoor cycling, you may find that you wander off the rollers and onto the floor, which can be quite a shock. Finally, mounting the rollers is easier with a friend's help.

Wind trainers work on a different principle. Most of these products require you to remove the front wheel of your bike and mount it onto the frame. The back wheel is then placed on rollers. A fan on the front, driven by the speed of your bicycle wheel on the rollers, creates a wind resistance, so you have resistance as you pedal. Obviously, the faster you go, the greater the resistance. Wind trainers, therefore, give good resistance, but balance and coordination development is minimal because the bicycle is attached to the wind trainer.

Most wind trainers have sealed fan bearings, a quick release fork attachment, and a bottom bracket support that adjusts for different sizes of bikes.

There is also a hybrid between these two products: a wind trainer with rollers only. A small fan on the back rollers provides resistance as you pedal.

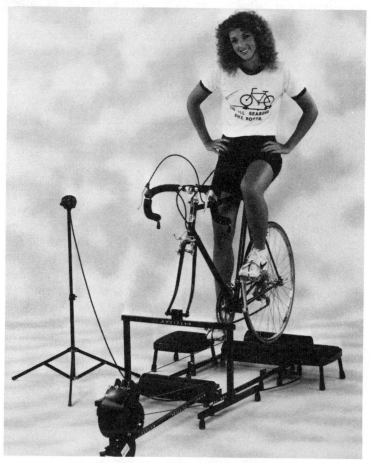

The Kreitler "Headwind" Wind Trainer

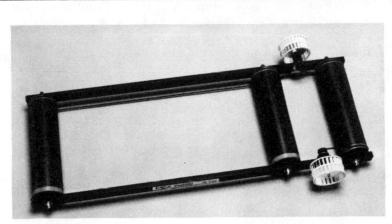

The Tacx Trainer   Photo courtesy of Tacx

ADVANTAGES AND DISADVANTAGES OF
EXERCISE BICYCLES AND ERGOMETERS

The general advantages of exercise bikes and ergometers are obvious. Both help you develop pedal action, burn calories, firm leg muscles, improve cardiovascular fitness, and maintain fitness throughout the year.

The main disadvantage of both is that the upper body is not exercised adequately. (There are a few exceptions; e.g., Schwinn AirDyne, which allows you to move the handlebars as you ride.) Also, since you are cycling indoors, the ride can be quite boring. So diversions such as stereo or TV may be necessary. (If you are serious about fitness and plan on exercising vigorously, reading and knitting are really not possible.)

It is also important to consider the specific advantages and disadvantages of the exercise bike and ergometer.

ADVANTAGES OF THE STATIONARY BIKE

- Stationary bicycles are less expensive than ergometers. They range from $59.95 to $300. Those that cost $225 or more are usually superior to the cheaper models.
- Exercise bicycles are less complicated to operate than ergometers. Since ergometers may use terms such as *kilopound meters*, *Newton meter*, and *watts*, the can be intimidating. The

exercise bicycle is a simple machine. Besides the frame, wheels, pedals, handlebars, and so forth, it has an odometer, speedometer, a device to program resistance, and a timer.
- Because of the simplicity of the stationary bicycle, it is usually easier to repair.
- There are more exercise bike dealers available than cycle ergometer dealers, so an exercise bike may be easier to buy.

ADVANTAGES OF THE ERGOMETER

- The first and most obvious advantage of an ergometer is that the work load can be calibrated. That means that if you have a specific health problem or are interested in improving your fitness for sport, the ergometer allows you to use a precise measure of resistance. In the beginning, calibration may not seem significant. But as you become more sophisticated and start to "fall in love" with indoor exercise, you may want some options that allow you to program the work load.

  Closely allied to the above is that, because an exercise bicycle lacks calibration, your selection of training plans is reduced. You must base your exercise on how you feel and on your pulse rate.
- An ergometer can also be used for testing. That is, you can compare yourself with others—family members or national norms. A doctor may use the ergometer for stress testing.
- An ergometer provides many more training options. If you are serious about training for triathlons, or you're using a bike for conditioning in the off-season, the ergometer gives you extra training plans.
- An ergometer allows you to calculate quickly the number of calories you use when exercising.
- Most cycle ergometers tend to be quieter than stationary bikes. The only way you can tell if the bike or ergometer is too noisy is to ride it before purchasing.

2

THE BENEFITS

THE MANY BENEFITS of indoor cycling include conditioning the heart, reducing body fat and/or weight, toning the leg muscles, and providing a mental "buzz."

Indoor cycling is basically an aerobic exercise. Aerobic exercise is exercise vigorous enough to burn a lot of calories, condition the heart, and improve the body's ability to transport oxygen throughout the body. It is not so vigorous, however, that it leaves the exerciser gasping and panting for breath.

IMPROVED HEART FITNESS

Your heart's job (and the blood vessels' job) is to send blood through your body quickly and efficiently. The blood carries oxygen to various sites to enable you to do certain tasks. Oxygen helps your muscles contract, your brain think, and your organs function. The blood also carries carbon dioxide (waste), which is eliminated so that your muscles, organs, and brain can continue to contract, function, and think, respectively. A regular exercise program on an indoor bicycle or ergometer will improve your body's ability to transport oxygen throughout your body. How?

Proper amounts of oxygen permit your cells and tissues to work in an efficient manner. Oxygen is delivered to your tissues by means of your heart, blood, and blood vessels. When you are fit, your circulatory system becomes more efficient. That means your aerobic capacity is improved. Regular aerobic exercise on a bicycle may provide these benefits:

1. Increase the number and size of your blood vessels for better and more efficient circulation.
2. Increase the elasticity of the blood vessels, thereby permitting more blood to circulate.
3. Increase the efficiency of exercising muscles and circulating blood so that muscles and blood are better able to pick up, carry, and use oxygen.
4. Increase the efficiency of the heart, allowing it to pump more blood with fewer beats.
5. Increase the number of red blood cells so that more oxygen can be carried throughout your body.

These five things, plus some other complicated biochemical changes over a period of weeks and months, permit your body to improve its ability to pick up, deliver, and use oxygen. The result is more oxygen available to the tissues. In turn, the bike riding becomes a lot easier.

Looking specifically at research on cycling and heart disease, the Netherlands Heart Foundation found that activities such as walking, cycling, and gardening without seasonal interruption lessen the risk of heart attack. The *British Medical Journal* also reported on the health of lifetime British cyclists over 50 years of age. These cyclists were members of the Fellowship of Cycling Old Timers. They had cycled 5,000–10,000 miles a year when younger and 2,000 miles a year more recently. Seventy-five percent of the 300 questioned still cycled at least once a week *throughout the year*. This group, compared to the general population, had fewer heart attacks and health problems. The 75-years-and-over group had 10 times less heart disease than the general population.

REDUCED BODY WEIGHT AND FAT

The fat cells of your body are your fuel storage tanks. When you burn off fewer calories through activity than your body takes in, you convert these extra calories into fat. This fat is then deposited in fat cells. To illustrate this point, suppose that you eat 2,400 calories' worth of food during a 24-hour period, and your level of activity is such that you burn off exactly 2,400 calories as you work, sleep, and play your way through the day. The supply and demand are equal. Your body neither calls on reserves to make up the energy deficit nor deposits extra calories in the form of fat. You maintain your weight. However, if you consume 2,400 calories and burn off only 2,300 of them, your body will convert those 100 unnecessary calories of food into fat and "store" it until such time as it's needed for energy.

One pound of fat is equivalent to 3,500 unnecessary calories. Whether these calories you eat are in the form of sirloin steak, ice cream, or raw carrots makes no difference. A calorie is a calorie. With this in mind, you can see that, if you eat 100 calories a day more than you burn off in physical activity, at the end of 35 days, you will have gained a pound. If you continue at the same rate, you will be 10 pounds heavier at the end of next year.

The reverse is also true. If you bicycle for three miles at your training heart rate, you'll burn 100 calories or so. Assuming you are now maintaining your weight, and you pedal three miles a day for 35 days, you'll lose 1 pound. In a year, the daily three-mile ride would amount to slightly more than 10 pounds lost.

When people lose weight merely by dieting, they often remain flabby. If you exercise while you diet or use exercise as the means for losing weight, your muscles become much firmer. Therefore, you will look and feel better after losing weight through exercise than you will after mere dieting.

The reason lies in an understanding of the fat-loss principle. Basically, there is one way to lose fat: establish a caloric deficit. That simply means that you burn off more calories than you eat. Of course, no one "eats" a calorie. We eat potatoes, meat, pies, and the rest, which contain units called calories. If the calories in these foods are not used, they are stored as fat. To lose extra poundage, you have two choices: decrease the amount of food you eat or increase the amount of calories you use.

FIRMED LEG MUSCLES

Cycling does more than reduce calories; it also tones and firms leg muscles. Let's look at the kinesiology of your body when bicycling.

There are four different muscular actions when pedaling. The first is the extension of the thigh at the hip joint. The thigh is extended at the hip joint with the aid of the gluteus maximus (buttocks muscle) and the adductor magnus (the muscle on the inside of the leg).

The second muscle action is the extension of the leg at the knee joint. This movement comes from the four sets of muscles on the front and outside of the thigh, known as the *quadriceps.*

The third action—extension of the foot at the ankle joint—is made possible by the gastrocnemius and soleus, the two muscles on the back of the calf.

The fourth and final action occurs when the leg is brought upward. If toe clips are used, the muscles on the front of the lower leg (tibialis anterior) are used. These muscles are helped by the quadriceps.

So the muscles and parts of the legs conditioned and strengthened through bicycling are the buttocks, thigh (inner, outer, and front), calf, and shin muscles. Coupled with the reduction in body fat because of the aerobic nature of bicycling, this conditioning gives your legs a form and shape that you thought were lost forever. Your buttocks become firmer and smaller. Your thighs go in where they are supposed to and out where they should. Your calves become well-defined in relation to the ankle.

Women who fear their calves will become larger through bicycling should consider this: Ride a bike and have small buttocks and well-developed, firmer, and yes, possibly larger calves. Or sit and watch TV, and you'll have a well-endowed buttocks area, smaller calves, and fatter ankles. The choice is yours.

MENTAL BENEFITS

Stress is prevalent. The frustration, anger, and hostilities you may feel could cause high blood pressure, headaches, and other stress ailments. How you deal with stressful situations is the important issue, and it is possible that a change in activity can help you master the feelings brought on by stress. The late Dr. Hans Selye, one of the world's foremost authorities on stress, stated that "stress on one system helps to relax the other." Here are some examples of how exercise, specifically aerobic exercise, including bicycling, can give you a mental lift.

ANGER AND ANXIETY ABATEMENT

Exercise can play an important role in helping to relieve anger and anxiety. Dr. William P. Morgan, researcher par excellence on emotions and exercise at the University of Wisconsin, noted at a recent conference that after a vigorous workout there is a measurable decrease in anxiety. The level of adrenaline in the blood, the blood pressure, and the heart rate are also reduced. Clinically, many people report improved feelings and less anxiety after a good bout of strenuous exercise.

While it is difficult at the present time to determine how exercise improves the mind and why it reduces anger and anxiety, it probably will be demonstrated in the future that the brain's nerve transmitters are changed in some way that causes people to feel better and more vigorous.

While I could continue to quote other people and studies on anxiety and anxiousness, I think Dr. Alan Clark of St. Joseph's Infirmary in Atlanta, Georgia, summarized it best: "It is well known that exercise is the best tranquilizer. I refuse to medicate patients with simple neurotic anxiety until they have given aerobic exercise an adequate trial." Amen!

DEPRESSION AND BLUES

Psychologists and psychiatrists are now looking at exercise as an option to help people handle the blues, or mild depression. For some reason, aerobic exercise seems to be a mood elevator. Studies done at the University of Virginia with students who claimed to suffer from depression showed that those who worked out vigorously three times a week for 10 weeks had an improvement in their scores on tests designed to measure depression. Working out lifted their feelings.

Such changes as raising a person out of depression, reducing anxiety, and transferring stress can make exercising addictive. People find that they need to exercise as much as others need their morning cup of coffee. According to Dr. William Glasser, physician and author of several books, exercise can transform negative addictions into positive ones. Those involved often choose to give up such things as smoking, drinking, overeating, and nonproductive arguing in favor of something more enjoyable and constructive—exercise.

OTHER ADVANTAGES

In addition to the potential heart fitness, fat loss, muscle and mental benefits, there are other advantages of indoor bicycle riding.

First, indoor bikes and ergometers are convenient. They may be placed in your favorite room or office, so exercise is only a step or two away. Furthermore, they may be ridden regardless of the weather. Closely allied to all of this is that the exercise bicycle is a constant reminder to you to exercise. That is especially important in the beginning stages of your exercise program.

Second, the indoor bike has several advantages over running. Since the exerciser's weight is supported by the bike or ergometer seat, fewer orthopedic problems arise. Therefore, the indoor bike is great for arthritics, the obese, and people with joint problems. Since ergometers can be calibrated and the work load established accurately, they are perfect for recovering heart attack victims.

I hate to admit it, but indoor bicycles also allow you to do two things at one time: exercise and watch TV, exercise and listen to music, even exercise and read a book, although if you are serious about exercising, reading is difficult. While exercise should be a diversion from your normal activities, some people feel exercise is necessary but "boring" or "a waste of time." The indoor exercise bike refutes that argument. Now two things can be done at once.

3

THE BEST EQUIPMENT

YOU PROBABLY ALREADY have an exercise bicycle at home, but there are a few things about your equipment that you may want to consider. Perhaps a new bike is in order, or you may want to ask your dealer to refine your bike a bit so your goal of fitness can be achieved more comfortably and efficiently.

Over the past few years I've written several articles on exercise equipment for *Consumer Digest* and *Consumer Guide*. I've had the opportunity to evaluate quite a few products. Also, *Bicycling Magazine* and *Consumer Report* have tested exercise bicycles. Here are some guidelines from these sources to help you achieve your fitness goal.

1. **An exercise bike should be sturdy and provide a smooth ride.** The two go together. If the bike you selected is a lightweight, with a spoked wheel (plastic or rubber tire) and an inexpensive frame, look out. When you pedal faster than 15 miles an hour, the bike may start to move. A speed of 20–25 mph may cause the bike to shimmy on the floor. In addition, the wheel has little weight, so when you pedal there is no wheel weight to keep the wheel moving continuously. Consequently, the pedals seem to stall as they reach the top and bottom of their rotation. There is no momentum to

carry them over the top. The result: a jerky motion and a bike that is difficult and aggravating to ride.

Spokes are also dangerous, especially if you have small children around. The best indoor exercise bikes have a flywheel made of heavy cast iron or are weighted in some way to encourage momentum.

In addition, you must ask yourself, "Will the bike frame and pedals hold my frame?" If you weigh 150 pounds or more, you should expect the pedals along with the frame to withstand some heavy stressors.

2. An exercise bike should have variable resistance. In the past five years, I haven't seen any bike without this feature (see photo). Thank goodness. Only variable resistance will progressively allow you to increase your work load so that your body will experience the training effect. Manufacturers have different methods of providing the resistance. Some bikes have a roller that rubs against the wheel. This is the least desirable resistance device. Others have caliper-type brakes (brake shoes) that exert pressure on the wheel as it turns (see photo). There are substantial differences in quality among the caliper or the brake shoe brakes. Some have small surface areas that wear away quickly. Others have broad surfaces that are up to the task of continuously providing resistance to the flywheel as it turns.

A third type of resistance uses a nylon strap. The strap is placed around the outside of the flywheel. Resistance is applied to the flywheel by tightening the nylon strap (see photo).

It's also important for the resistance dial to be within easy reach—on the handlebar or on the frame. That way you can increase the resistance while pedaling vigorously. Second, the dial should provide a variety of settings. Stay away from those that provide only two settings—hard and easy.

3. An exercise bike should have a seat and handlebars that are adjustable. If you can't lower and raise the seat and handlebars, you may be headed for trouble (see photo). The seat is the more important of the two. Optimally, it will be self-adjusting (no wrench is needed). It's also best if it can be changed to the point where the distance from the seat to the lowest pedal position is equal to your crotch-to-floor measurement plus two inches. This allows room for you to extend your foot when pedaling, if you so desire.

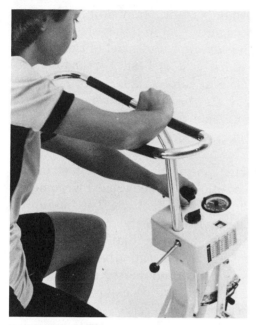

The Bodyguard 900, with variable resistance.

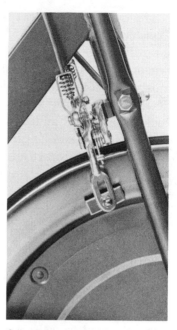

Caliper-type brakes

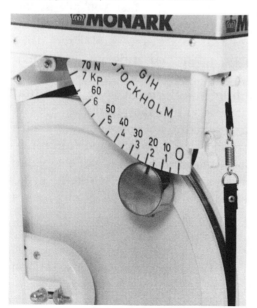

The nylon strap at right creates necessary resistance.

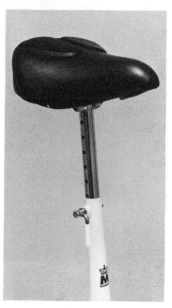

It's important that you adjust the bike seat to fit your height and leg reach.

The quality of the seat is also important. Many people who ride exercise bikes complain of a sore butt. And well they should. Some manufacturers cheat on this highly important part of the bike. A reasonably wide and well-padded seat is best. Fortunately, on most models an inferior bicycle seat can be replaced by a better-designed seat. The seat should also be rigid. You don't want it rocking forward and back, and side to side, as you pedal. This rocking action can be quite aggravating.

It's also good to have adjustable handlebars (see photo). I like the flexibility of having them upright in the classic position or in the drop-bar "racing or training" position. The Bodyguard Ergometer 990 model has this feature, which is a real delight. The flexibility to adjust the bars higher or lower gives greater comfort during long exercise bouts. I will admit, however, that the handlebar height adjustment is not as crucial as the seat adjustment.

4. An exercise bike should have an odometer and a speedometer. Odometers and speedometers are necessary for motivation and minimum quantification of exercise (see photo). At present, most exercise bikes have both. These products are good motivators—they tell you how far and how fast you are going. They also allow you to measure progress made—miles traveled, miles per hour—compared to training heart rate. From this, calories expended can be calculated and mileage on a map plotted—all good motivational factors.

5. Pedals on the exercise bike should meet your individual needs. Most people prefer broad, smooth pedals similar to those on a regular outdoor bicycle. Many bikes do not come equipped with these. However, you can ask your distributor to provide appropriate pedals. Also, I prefer a cloth strap across the top of the pedal. Called a *stirrup* or *toe clip*, this allows a pulling action on the pedal as you bring your leg up from its down position. The toe clip makes for more efficient pedaling (see photo).

6. A stationary bicycle should be quiet. A noisy bike is usually a sign of poor construction and improperly fitted parts. You'll want a quiet machine for two important reasons: (1) You don't want to bother someone else. (2) You may want to listen to music as you ride. Noisy bikes are a real distraction.

7. You should be comfortable on your exercise bike. In regular bicycling, position is basic, according to James C. McCullagh, editor and publisher of *Bicycling Magazine*. The same is true

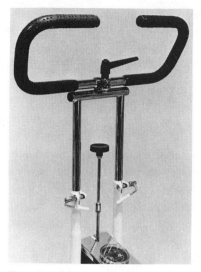

These handlebars can be adjusted both horizontally and vertically.

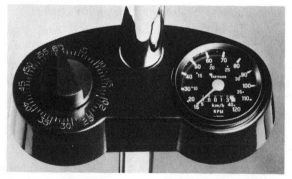

Your bike should have a speedometer, odometer, and timer.

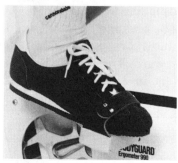

A broad pedal with a toe stirrup will give you the best control.

of stationary bicycling. So here are some guidelines to make your exercise more enjoyable and less fatiguing. The key is proper positioning. These recommendations are based largely on McCullagh's excellent book, *The Complete Bicycle Fitness Book*. His notes are for the regular cyclist. I have adapted them for the indoor exercise bicycle.

Saddle Height. Most novices start on their exercise bicycle with the seat too low. Unfortunately, when the seat is in this position, your legs are bent too much. This position does not allow you to use your legs as efficiently as possible. They cramp up more easily, and the exchange of oxygen and carbon dioxide is not as efficient as it could be. The second mistake is to raise the seat too high. Somewhere, people have heard that the legs should be fully extended at the bottom of the pedal stroke.

Quite frankly, an in-between position is best. That is, place your saddle at a height so that when you put your heels on the pedals you can pedal freely without having to rock your buttocks from side to side to reach the bottom of the pedal stroke.

Foot Position. The ball of your foot should be on top of the pedal, preferably directly on top of the pedal spindle. Avoid pedaling with the arch on the pedal. Toe clips or straps are desirable. Be sure they are positioned in such a way as to keep the ball of your foot on the pedal spindle. This position allows you to maximize the action of your calf muscles (gastrocnemius and soleus).

Saddle Position. The tilt of your saddle is very important. As McCullagh says, "A saddle with the nose too high will be uncomfortable in some mighty personal areas." If the nose is too low, you will always be leaning into the handlebars. Generally, the saddle should be *directly* parallel to the floor when first starting. You can adjust it after several weeks if it doesn't seem right for you.

Besides the tilt of the saddle, the distance of the saddle from the handlebars is important. Most people place the saddle too far forward. The best and simplest rule is to adjust the saddle so that it is in the middle of the seat post clamp. Then adjust the handlebar height to accommodate your reach.

If you want to be scientific, follow McCullagh's guidelines:

> You need a friend and a plumbline. Get on the bike in the riding position. . . . Put one pedal in the 3:00 (facing forward) position. Have your friend drop the plumbline from the bump on the top of your tibia (shinbone). (This bump is just below the kneecap.) The plumbline should fall to the ball of your foot, which is in position directly over the pedal spindle.

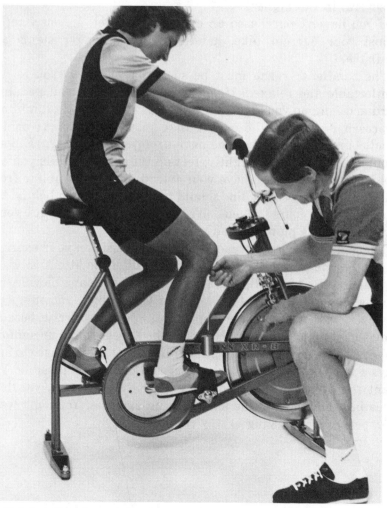

The McCullagh Plumbline technique makes it easy to determine the proper saddle height.

Handlebar Position. Handlebar height is a matter of personal preference and comfort, but the distance between you and the handlebars—the handlebar reach—is not.

If you are going to pedal hard and fast, you will probably prefer the handlebar height rather low, that is, several inches below the saddle level. That may not feel comfortable at first—so give it time.

If you prefer the height higher, move it up, especially if your back rebels to the low-slung position or if you are watching the 6 o'clock news. Here, the height may be level with the saddle height or several inches higher.

If you haven't purchased an exercise bike yet, or you want to adjust your current bike, handlebars with longer stems are available.

The handlebar reach must be such that it allows you to feel comfortable and relaxed. If you're really serious about pedaling hard and long on your bike, McCullagh's "friend and plumbline" approach is best. While on the bike, place your hands on the handlebars. I'm assuming you have dropped handlebars. Elbows should be bent ever so slightly, feet on the pedals. While you are looking straight ahead, have your friend drop a plumbline from the tip of your nose. The line should land one-half inch behind the handlebars. Of course, if you don't have dropped handlebars, you'll have to skip the plumbline adjustment.

That's it! You are now ready to train seriously on your exercise bicycle. Some of you may wonder about all of the attention we've paid to detail. After all, you are riding a stationary bicycle, not tooling down Main Street or around a Velodrome. I'm convinced, however, that many people stop indoor bicycle exercise because they hurt (particularly in the back or the knees) or feel uncomfortable. If you're going to spend 20–40 minutes on a bike three to four days a week, you want to make it as comfortable as possible. You want the bike to "feel good" to your body. After all, you'll be sweating enough from the leg-churning exercise. You don't want to expend energy trying to stay comfortable.

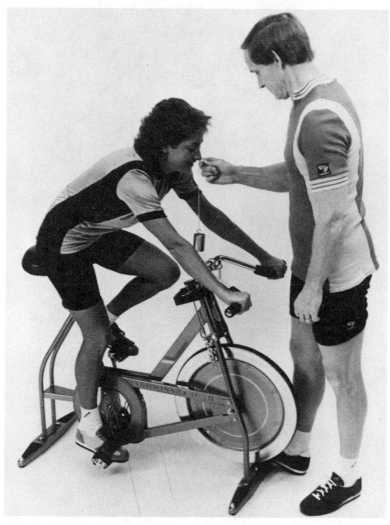

The McCullagh Plumbline technique also shows how to measure for correct handlebar position.

4

WORKING OUT

IN THIS CHAPTER, basic training regimens are provided for both the exercise bike and the cycle ergometer. These programs focus on continuous aerobic exercise based on your heart rate.

These workouts are designed for normal, healthy individuals. If you have a significant health problem—asthma, heart disease, high blood pressure, etc.—see Chapter 7. To use indoor bicycling as an adjunct to your sports training, see Chapter 6. Chapter 5 provides a training program for the cycle ergometer, utilizing the various resistance and calibrations available on this equipment.

Before you begin exercising, a word of caution is in order. If you have any question about your health and have not exercised in the past five years, check with your doctor. That is common sense. By the way, even if you don't plan on exercising and you have a question about your health, see your doctor. Your doctor can tell you whether you can afford to take that risk.

Also before training, you should know something about how hard, how long, and how often you should exercise for fitness benefits.

HOW MUCH EXERCISE DO YOU NEED?

The amount of exercise you need depends on personal goals and how you perceive your exercise. Basically, physiologists talk about intensity (how hard you exercise), duration (how long), and frequency (how often). Of these three factors, most experts favor intensity as the key factor in effective exercise, that is, getting your heart rate up to 130 beats per minute (or so) and keeping it there for 20–30 minutes. They also recommend exercising three times a week.

While these recommendations are valid, they do not take into account that the intensity may be decreased if the duration and frequency are increased. In other words, there is an interaction among these three factors. In reality, intensity, duration, and frequency make up a fourth factor—total work. Total work is the real key to fitness and weight control.

Let me explain. The most important factor in exercise is total work, that is, a combination of how hard, how long, and how often you exercise. Yes, a minimum heart rate threshold (somewhere between 40 and 50 percent of maximum), a minimum number of minutes (about 15–20 minutes), and a minimum number of days per week (two to four) are necessary for training. These factors can be adjusted, however, so that, if you work harder (more intensely), you do not need to exercise as long. But the converse is also true. If you work at lower intensity, you need to exercise longer. The charts in this book and the following discussions of how hard, how long, and how often you should exercise are based on this concept.

HOW HARD?

The best way to determine how hard you should exercise is to measure the maximum amount of oxygen your body is capable of using. To do this, doctors have you ride a specialized bicycle or walk or run on a treadmill. While you give it an all-out effort, the doctor measures the amount of oxygen you use. Since it is a maximum effort, it is called a *maximum oxygen uptake (max VO$_2$)*. With this information, the physician can give you a prescription for exercise intensity.

Most of us can't, or prefer not to, spend the required amount of money on this type of testing. Fortunately, there is an alternative:

HEART RATE

The number of times your heart pumps blood each minute is your pulse rate or heart rate. To feel your pulse, turn the palm of your hand up and place two or three fingers of your right hand on the thumb side of your left wrist. This point is called the *radial pulse*.

When taking your pulse, you should feel a push or thump against your fingers. Each push is one beat of your heart. This beat is called your *pulse*. The number of pushes each minute is your heart or pulse rate. If you have trouble locating your radial pulse, place your first two fingers on one side of your throat just below the point of the jaw and locate the carotid artery. As you do this, press lightly. Avoid pressing too hard when checking a carotid pulse.

After locating your heartbeat, look at the sweep second hand on your watch. Starting with zero, count the number of beats for a 10-second interval. Multiply that number by six. This represents your resting heart rate per minute.

Table 1:
Maximum Heart Rate

Age	Maximum Heart Rate (bpm)*
20	200
25	195
30	190
35	185
40	180
45	175
50	170
55	165
60	160
65	155
70	150

*bpm = beats per minute

checking your heart rate. When you exercise, your muscles demand more oxygen. Your heart rate and breathing speed up to send more oxygen to your exercising muscles. As you might expect, there is a parallel increase in heart rate and oxygen usage. Because of this parallel increase, you can use your heart rate as a worthy substitute for the sophisticated testing. Simply reach for your wrist and count your heartbeat (see box). Then make sure you exercise at a level that keeps your heart beating at the proper rate. That rate will be different for different people.

Everyone has a maximum heart rate. Your maximum heart rate is the number of beats your heart makes per minute when you are exercising as far, as fast, and as long as possible. Although it varies from person to person, your maximum heart rate is roughly 220 minus your age. If you are a 20-year-old, your maximum heart rate is about 20. If you are 40, it's about 180. (See Table 1.)

Do not try to exercise at your maximum heart rate. That is not necessary for general fitness. A safe and more appropriate level ranges between 40 and 75 percent of your maximum. That is your ideal heart rate range.

To find your ideal heart rate range, you must first find your resting heart rate. When you are rested, relaxed, and sitting or lying down, check your pulse for one minute to find your resting heart rate. Subtract the number of resting beats per minute from your maximum heart rate (see Table 1 above). That gives you your heart rate range. Then take 40–75 percent of this heart rate range and add that answer to your resting heart rate. For example, the calculation for a 40-year-old who has a resting heart rate of 60 will look like this:

$$
\begin{array}{rl}
180 & \text{Maximum heart rate} \\
\underline{-60} & \text{Resting heart rate} \\
120 & \text{Heart rate range}
\end{array}
$$

$$120 \times .40 = 48 + \text{Resting heart rate } (60) = 108$$
$$120 \times .75 = 90 + \text{Resting heart rate } (60) = 150$$

This person's ideal heart rate range would be 108–150 beats per minute.

To spare you from all this mathematical razzmatazz, simply look at the following tables, tables 2–7, in which all the calculations have been done for you. First, locate the table applicable to your age. Then find your resting heart rate at the top of your age table. From this you'll be able to find your ideal heart rate range for exercise.

Table 2:
Exercise Heart Rate Age 20 and Under

% of Max. Heart Rate	Resting Heart Rates					
	54 or less	55–64	65–74	75–84	85–94	95 or more
40%	110–115	116–122	122–127	128–133	134–139	140–144
45%	116–122	123–129	128–134	134–139	140–144	145–149
50%	123–129	130–136	135–141	140–145	145–149	150–154
55%	130–136	137–141	142–147	146–151	150–155	155–159
60%	137–143	142–147	148–153	152–157	156–161	160–164
65%	144–150	148–153	154–157	158–161	162–164	165–170
70%	151–156	154–160	158–162	162–165	165–168	169–174
75%	157–163	161–166	163–168	166–171	169–173	175–179

Table 3:
Exercise Heart Rate Age 20–29

% of Max. Heart Rate	Resting Heart Rates					
	54 or less	55–64	65–74	75–84	85–94	95 or more
40%	106–111	112–116	118–122	124–128	130–134	136–140
45%	112–118	117–123	123–128	129–134	135–140	141–145
50%	119–125	124–130	129–135	135–140	141–145	146–150
55%	126–132	131–137	136–142	141–146	146–150	151–155
60%	133–140	138–144	143–148	147–152	151–156	156–160
65%	141–148	145–151	149–154	153–158	157–162	161–165
70%	149–153	152–156	155–159	159–162	163–166	166–170
75%	154–160	157–162	160–165	163–167	167–170	171–175

Table 4:
Exercise Heart Rate Age 30–39

% of Max. Heart Rate	Resting Heart Rates					
	54 or less	55–64	65–74	75–84	85–94	95 or more
40%	102–106	108–112	114–118	120–124	126–130	132–136
45%	107–113	113–118	119–124	125–130	131–135	137–140
50%	114–120	119–125	125–130	131–135	136–140	141–145
55%	121–127	126–132	131–136	136–140	141–145	146–150
60%	128–134	133–138	137–142	141–146	146–150	151–154
65%	135–141	139–144	143–148	147–152	151–155	155–158
70%	142–146	145–149	149–152	153–155	156–158	158–161
75%	147–152	150–155	153–157	156–160	159–162	162–164

Table 5:
Exercise Heart Rate Age 40–49

% of Max. Heart Rate	Resting Heart Rates					
	54 or less	55–64	65–74	75–84	85–94	95 or more
40%	98–102	104–108	110–114	116–120	122–126	128–132
45%	103–108	109–114	115–120	121–125	127–130	133–136
50%	109–115	115–120	121–125	126–130	131–135	137–140
55%	116–122	121–126	126–130	131–135	136–140	141–144
60%	123–128	127–132	131–136	136–140	141–144	145–148
65%	129–134	133–138	137–142	141–145	145–148	149–152
70%	135–140	139–144	143–148	146–150	149–153	153–156
75%	141–145	145–150	149–154	151–155	154–158	159–162

To use these tables when riding an exercise bicycle, check your pulse after you have cycled for at least 10 minutes. During this ride, you should push yourself, but not too hard. You should be breathing more deeply than usual and will probably perspire. The exercise should be pain-free, you should be able to talk to someone next to you (real or imagined), and the bicycling pace should seem just about right.

Check your pulse for six seconds and multiply the number by 10 to determine your heart's beats per minute while exercising. Then

Table 6:
Exercise Heart Rate Age 50–59

% of Max. Heart Rate	Resting Heart Rates					
	54 or less	55–64	65–74	75–84	85–94	95 or more
40%	94– 98	100–104	106–110	112–116	118–122	124–128
45%	99–104	105–110	111–115	117–120	123–126	129–132
50%	105–110	111–115	116–120	121–125	127–130	133–135
55%	111–116	116–120	121–125	126–130	131–134	136–138
60%	117–122	121–126	126–130	131–134	135–138	139–142
65%	123–128	127–131	131–135	135–138	139–142	143–145
70%	129–132	132–135	136–139	139–141	143–145	146–148
75%	133–137	136–140	140–143	142–145	146–148	149–152

Table 7:
Exercise Heart Rate Age 60 and Above

% of Max. Heart Rate	Resting Heart Rates					
	54 or less	55–64	65–74	75–84	85–94	95 or more
40%	89– 94	96–100	102–106	109–112	115–118	122–124
45%	95–100	101–105	107–111	113–116	119–122	125–127
50%	101–106	106–110	112–115	117–120	123–125	128–130
55%	107–111	111–116	116–120	121–124	126–129	131–134
60%	112–117	117–121	121–125	125–129	130–133	135–137
65%	118–122	122–126	126–129	130–133	134–136	138–140
70%	123–126	125–130	128–132	132–137	135–140	141–144
75%	127–130	131–133	133–136	138–140	140–144	145–148

locate your resting heart rate column (across the top) and find your pulse in the vertical column. Look at the far left column for the percentage of maximum heart rate (fitness category). Remember that category. You'll need it in the following section. You'll notice that our 40-year-old has a range of 108–150 on the chart just as he or she did in the calculation given earlier. If your heart rate is higher than the range provided, slow down your cycling pace. If your heart rate is lower than the range provided, pick up your pace a bit during the next exercise session.

HOW LONG?

When you are exercising to train your heart and lungs, most experts agree that at least 20 minutes of exercise at 60–65 percent of heart rate range is necessary. My research generally agrees with that. I have also found that the intensity may be increased or decreased, but more on that in a minute.

When you are exercising to burn calories and fat efficiently, most experts agree that at least 300 kilocalories (calories) should be burned or used when exercising to help control your body weight. (Experts use the number of calories burned during exercise as a measure of total work.) Usually one-half hour of exercise is recommended with the heart rate being at about 60 percent of your heart rate range.

There are several reasons for these 300 calories or one-half hour. At rest, the majority of your energy comes from glycogen and glucose (carbohydrate). As you exercise, your body gradually shifts into burning fat stores. The longer you exercise, the more fat you use. Exercising for 30 minutes (or burning 300 calories) seems to be the critical threshold you must reach to burn away fat and keep it off.

Of course, some people cannot burn 300 calories in one-half hour. They find the 60-percent exercise range too difficult, so they want to back off a bit on the intensity. They find that exercising at 40 percent of their heart rate for 60 minutes is more comfortable. This level of exercise for 60 minutes still burns 300 calories.

Not everyone is able to exercise at the 60-percent level of intensity. For them, 40 or 50 percent may be better or more comfortable. Therefore, they must exercise longer to adjust for the reduced intensity. Table 8 shows you how long to exercise, based on pulse rates. When you are cycling, check your pulse and determine your percentage of maximum heart rate as described above. You are now able to determine the number of minutes you should exercise.

For example, if you are riding and your heart rate is at 60 percent of maximum, you should ride for 30–37½ minutes; if you are riding at 50 percent of your maximum heart rate, you'll need to cycle for 45–52½ minutes. Cycling at 75 percent of your maximum heart rate is necessary for only 15–20 minutes. When you exercise at these heart rates for the specified duration, you will burn or use 300 calories.

Table 8:
Number of Minutes of Recommended Exercise
at Different Training Heart Rates

% of Maximum Heart Rate	Number of Minutes to Exercise— Fat/Weight Control	Number of Minutes to Exercise— Heart/Lung Fitness
40%	60:01–75:00	Not Intense Enough
45%	52:31–60:00	Not Intense Enough
50%	45:01–52:30	45:01–52:30
55%	37:30–45:00	37:30–45:00
60%	30:01–37:30	30:01–37:30
65%	25:01–30:00	25:01–30:00
70%	20:01–25:00	20:01–25:00
75%	15:00–20:00	15:00–20:00

Just to make sure you've got it, let's review: There is a strong interplay between the intensity and duration of exercise, that is, how long and how hard you exercise. You may lower the intensity of your exercise by exercising for longer periods of time, or you may work at a higher intensity for a shorter duration. Specifically, if you want to improve your heart and lung fitness, the ideal way is to exercise for 30–37½ minutes at a heart rate of 60 percent of your heart rate range. If you find, however, that the 60-percent range is too difficult or leaves you breathless, then exercise at 50 percent of your heart rate range for 45–52½ minutes. On the other hand, if you find 60 percent too easy, you may work at 70–75 percent of maximum and exercise for 15–20 minutes. Regardless, the goal is to burn 300 calories.

HOW OFTEN?

Ride a minimum of three to five times a week. Studies show that exercising this many times a week provides a reasonable and optimum frequency of exercise. Once you are fit, two to three times a week may help you maintain your fitness level, but three and preferably four or five times is best for getting into shape, losing fat, and staying lean over the long haul.

Make sure you understand the relationship of how hard, how long, and how often you need to exercise. I'm going to come back to it later.

THE BASIC TRAINING:
EXERCISE BIKE AND CYCLE ERGOMETER

The basic training program is broken down into three phases: the warm-up, peak work, and the cool-down. The warm-up is approximately 10 minutes long, the peak work is 15–75 minutes (depending on your goal), and the cool-down is 10 minutes. The warm-up is designed to get your body ready for more vigorous exercise. Since you have been sedentary, you need to loosen joints; stretch muscles, tendons, and ligaments; and prepare the cardiovascular system for more demanding exercise. Then you are ready to move into the peak period. The cool-down does the reverse—prepares your body for the sedentary lifestyle. Let's look at each aspect.

THE WARM-UP: 10 MINUTES

Before you get on the bike, spend a few minutes doing the following exercises. Since your body temperature will not be elevated at this point, your muscles will be "cold," and you probably will not be able to stretch adequately. Therefore, these exercises are viewed as joint mobility exercises.

Knee Raises
1. Lie on your back with your legs bent.
2. Hold your right knee with both hands and pull it toward your chest. Hold for 10 seconds, relax, and return to the original position.
3. Repeat with the left knee. Do this exercise three times.

Bike Quadriceps Stretch
1. Stand beside a bike, holding on to it with your left hand.
2. Put your weight on your left leg, bend your right leg and hold on to your right ankle with your right hand.
3. Pull your right thigh back, keeping your left leg straight. Concentrate on relaxing the muscles. As the muscles relax, stretch even further to the point of a "tug." Hold for 10 seconds, then relax.

After doing these preliminary exercises, get on your bike and ride for five minutes at a minimum resistance (that is, so it feels as if you are pedaling on an even surface outdoors). Pedal at 80–90

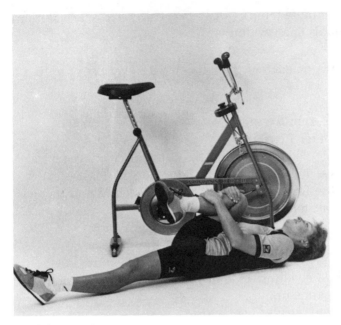

Knee Raises

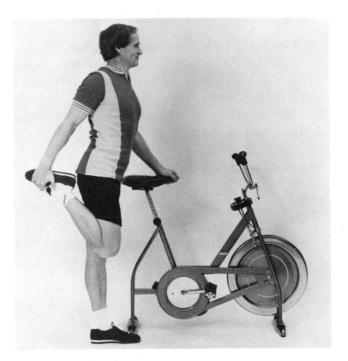

Bike Quadriceps Stretch

revolutions per minute (rpm). One turn or downstroke (revolution) for *each* leg equals one revolution.

While pedaling, do each of the following 12 exercises for 15–20 seconds.

Alternate High Arm Swings

Improves shoulder flexibility.

1. Sitting while pedaling, swing the arms alternately forward and backward. The hands should reach at least shoulder height on the forward swing. You can reach higher as your program continues.

Arm Circles

Good for the deltoid muscle, which caps the shoulder.

1. Sitting while pedaling, extend your arms straight out at the shoulders, palms up.
2. Describe small circles backward.
3. Then turn the palms down and circle in the opposite direction.

Arm Flex (Arm Flexion and Extension)

Helps tone both the biceps and the triceps muscles.

1. Sitting while pedaling, extend your arms to the sides at shoulder height. Palms should be up.
2. Then flex the arms inward as though making a muscle.
3. Then extend the arms.

Arms above the Head and Shoulders

Helps return blood to the heart.

1. Sitting while pedaling, stretch your arms above the shoulders and shake them easily.

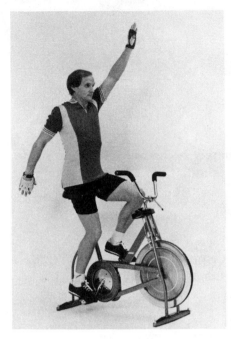

Alternate High Arm Swings

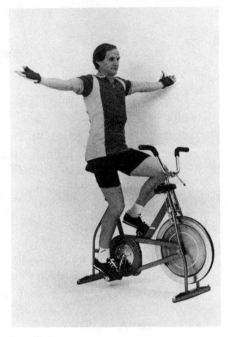

Arm Circles

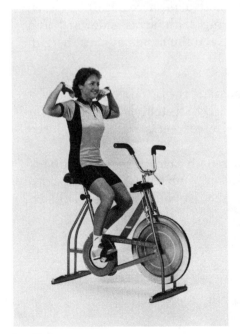

Arm Flex

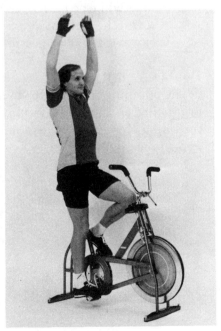

Arms above the head and shoulders

Backward Crawl

Improves shoulder flexibility.

1. Sitting while pedaling, alternately swing your arms upward, backward, and around, simulating the swimming backstroke.

Boxer

Helps tone both the triceps and biceps muscles.

1. Sitting while pedaling, simulate punching a punching bag by beginning with the arms extended, then drawing them back in front of the body, then moving them from left to right.

Cross-Body Arm Swings

Helps to prevent or correct a round-shouldered appearance.

1. Sitting while pedaling, swing both arms across the body, then reverse the action by swinging both arms sideward and backward as far as possible. Keep the hands at chest height.

Double-Arm Pumps

The pumping action helps to massage the blood vessels, thereby promoting circulatory stimulation. By stretching the muscles of the chest, this exercise also helps to correct a round-shouldered appearance.

1. Sitting while pedaling, swing both arms forward and back simultaneously along the sides of your body. On the forward swings, flex both arms, draw the fist in toward the shoulders, and pump twice.

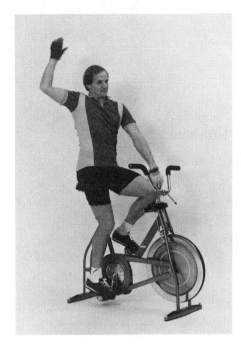

Backward Crawl

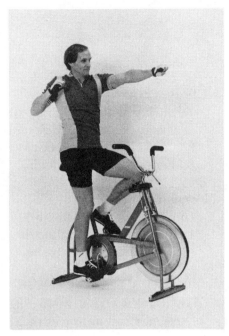

Boxer

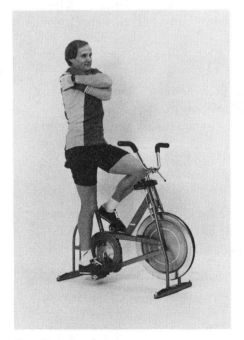

Cross-Body Arm Swings

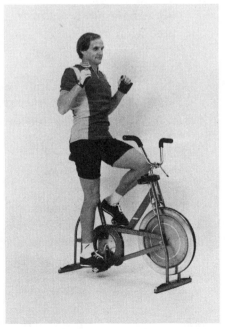

Double Arm Pumps

Elbow Circles

1. Sitting while pedaling, place your right hand on the right shoulder and your left on the left shoulder.
2. Circle both elbows clockwise.
3. Repeat counterclockwise.

Forward Crawl

Improves shoulder flexibility.

1. Sitting while pedaling, let the arms hang relaxed. Swing the right and left arms alternately backward, upward, and forward, simulating the swimming crawl stroke.

Giant Backward Arm Circles

Stretches and improves the flexibility of the chest and shoulder muscles.

1. Sitting while pedaling, swing the arms in a complete circle, upward and across in front of the body and then backward and around.

Arm Flings

1. Sitting while pedaling, bend your arms at the elbows, with hands held in loose fists at chest height.
2. Push both elbows backward, then return to the starting position.
3. Straighten the arms and fling them backward, then return to the starting position.

After doing these warm-up exercises, check your pulse rate. Your heart rate should be increased. At this point, you are ready to move into the peak work load phase.

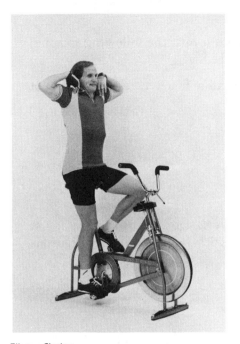

Elbow Circles

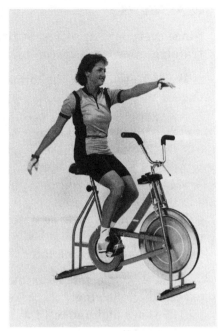

Forward Crawl

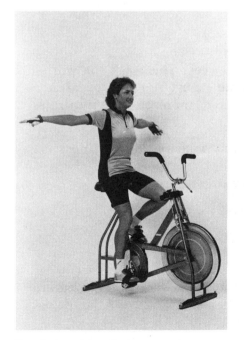

Giant Backward Arm Circles

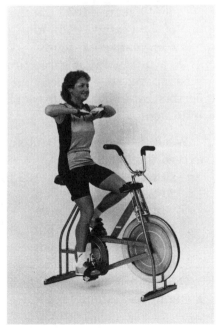

Arm Flings

PEAK WORK

Since everyone has different fitness levels, the following gradual training approach is recommended.

Week 1. Cycle for 10 minutes at a heart rate that does not exceed the following:

    20 years and under—115 bpm
    20–29 years—110 bpm
    30–39 years—105 bpm
    40–49 years—100 bpm
    50–59 years—100 bpm
    60+ years—95 bpm

Do a minimum of three times a week. Do not push yourself; just ride to condition your body to withstand the more vigorous exercise that will come later.

Week 2. Cycle for 15 minutes at a heart rate that does not exceed the following:

    20 years and under—120 bpm
    20–29 years—115 bpm
    30–39 years—110 bpm
    40–49 years—105 bpm
    50–59 years—105 bpm
    60+ years—100 bpm

Do a minimum of three times a week. This week you will be pushing yourself harder, but again, don't strive to pedal at a certain rate. Just try to work so you approach the pulse rates indicated.

Week 3. Cycle for 20 minutes at a heart rate that does not exceed the following:

    20 years and under—125 bpm
    20–29 years—120 bpm
    30–39 years—115 bpm
    40–49 years—110 bpm
    50–59 years—110 bpm
    60+ years—105 bpm

Do a minimum of three to four times a week. Again, you are going to be pushing yourself a little harder this week, but do not exceed those pulse rates.

Week 4. Cycle for 25 minutes at a heart rate that does not exceed the following:

20 years and under—130 bpm

20-29 years—125 bpm

30-39 years—120 bpm

40-49 years—115 bpm

50-59 years—115 bpm

60+ years—110 bpm

Do a minimum of four times a week. This four-week preparation plan will get your cardiovascular system and leg muscles ready for some demanding exercise.

In the event that your body doesn't seem ready for more demanding exercise, stay at Week 4 level for several more weeks until your body calls for more demanding exercise.

Weeks 5 and On. Now you are ready to get into the swing of things. Your legs and cardiovascular system should be ready to handle your ideal heart rate range. You are now ready to go back to the principles we talked about on pages 28–35.

On the first day of exercise of the fifth week, go through your normal warm-up for 10 minutes. After the warm-up, cycle for at least 10 minutes. During this ride, push yourself, but not too hard. You should be breathing more deeply than when at rest, your heart rate should be higher, and you should be perspiring. The exercise should be pain-free and you should be able to talk to someone next to you (real or imaginary). You should also feel as though you could go at least another 20 minutes at this exercise level. And finally, the exercise should seem just right—exhilarating.

Stop after 10 minutes and *immediately* check your pulse for six seconds. Take that figure and multiply the number by 10 to determine your heart rate when exercising. Then go to Tables 2-7. Locate your resting heart rate column (across the top) and find your exercise pulse in the vertical column. After you have located your exercise heart rate, look at the far left column for the percentage of maximum heart rate. In table 9, on the following page, is an example for a 40-year-old with a resting heart rate of 70 and a just-completed exercise heart rate of 135. He or she is working at 60 percent of the maximum heart rate.

Table 9:
Sample Heart Rate Figures

% of Heart Rate	Resting HR = 70
40%	110–114
45%	115–120
50%	121–125
55%	126–130
60%	131–136
65%	137–142
70%	143–148
75%	149–154

Once you have your percentage of maximum heart rate, turn to Table 8 on page 35. If your goal is to improve heart/lung fitness or control your body fat, pedal for 30–37½ minutes at this heart rate. My suggestion is to start on the low side (about 30 minutes) and, over the next few weeks, perhaps three or four, improve to where you can pedal for 37:30.

The number of days you should exercise depends on your goal: cardiovascular fitness or weight and fitness control. If it's cardiovascular fitness, three times a week is the minimum. For weight control and fitness, four times a week is your minimum.

So, using the 40-year-old female as an example, exercising for weight and figure control, she should exercise at a heart rate range of 131–136 beats per minute (60 percent of maximum) four times a week. By the way, the exercise should be done every other day: Monday/Wednesday/Friday/Sunday or Tuesday/Thursday/Saturday/Monday. Avoid exercising on succeeding days.

Stick with this exercise intensity daily. Record the miles per hour you pedaled and the distance covered. Keep a diary. In the Appendix of this book, you will find space for recording the information. These daily records will give a measure of improvement or lack of improvement, so you can monitor your progress. The idea is to cover more miles in the same length of time without a corresponding increase in exercise pulse rate.

Over the weeks, your fitness level and tolerance to exercise will improve. Every four weeks you should retest yourself. After warm-up, ride for 10 minutes and, at a rate that seems right for you, check your pulse and redefine your workout rate.

Most people will stay at the same level (percentage of heart rate) except those who were below 55 percent of maximum heart rate level. As the weeks progress, and they get into better shape, they are usually able to tolerate greater work loads, so they increase their exercise intensity. Therefore, the more fit you become and the higher level of exercise you are able to do, the fewer minutes you may spend exercising. This apparent paradox is explained by the total work phenomenon defined earlier. Working at 55 percent of your maximum heart rate for 45 minutes uses the same amount of energy as working at 65 percent of your maximum heart rate for 30 minutes. Each combination of intensity and duration shown in Table 8 will cause you to expend 300 calories.

COOL-DOWN: 10 MINUTES

After your peak work phase, it is time to cool down. The heart cool-down phase should proceed as follows: Spend five minutes after the peak work pedaling slower at a decreased resistance on your variable resistance dial. Allow your body to recover. Sudden stopping may cause some light-headedness, so pedal at a lower resistance and at a slower pace—maybe one-half to three-quarters of what you have been pedaling. For example, if you have been pedaling at 25 miles per hour, you should slow down to 12–20 mph. If you were pedaling at a resistance of three, during the cool-down a one would be appropriate.

After the five minutes of easy cycling, stop pedaling and do the following stretches. With all these stretches, stretch to the point where you feel a "tug." Hold that position and, while relaxing, visualize the muscles that are being stretched. When they do loosen up, go to the point of a second tug, hold that position for 10 seconds, and return. Over the weeks, gradually increase your hold time to 30 seconds.

Sitting Side Stream
1. While sitting on the bike, place both hands above the head, outstretched as high as possible. Clasp your hands together.
2. Bend to the right, keeping the hands clasped together, and hold.
3. Return to the starting position and repeat to the left.
4. Repeat to both sides again.

Sitting Tiptoes
1. While sitting on the bike, raise your right leg so that it is parallel to the floor. (You may need to adjust the handlebar location.)
2. Point your toes away from you and hold.
3. Then pull the toes toward the knees or shin and hold.
4. Repeat for the left side.

Sitting Hands Up
1. While sitting on the bike, place your hands at your sides with the palms facing backward.
2. From this position, keeping your arms straight, raise both arms back and up toward the ceiling. Hold.
3. Return to the starting position and repeat.

Single-Leg Tucks
Stretches the muscles at the back of your thigh (hamstrings) as well as the lower back.
1. Sit on the floor with your left leg straight and your right leg bent. Tuck your right foot into the groin.
2. Bend from the waist, reach forward, and clasp your left ankle. Pull your chest toward your left knee. Hold.
3. Repeat with the right leg.

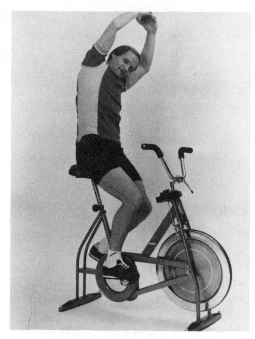

Sitting Side Stream

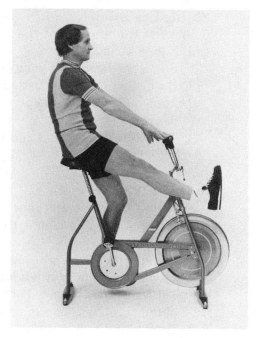

Sitting Tiptoes

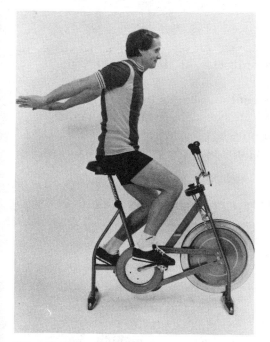

Sitting Hand-Up

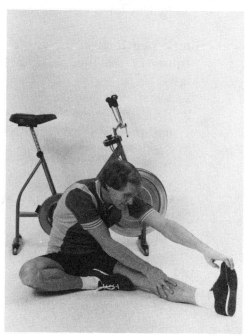

Single Leg Tuck

Sitting Leg Stretch

Benefits the muscles of the lower back and those behind the thighs (hamstrings).

1. Sit on the floor with your legs extended.
2. Bend slowly at the waist and bring your head as close to the knees as possible. Keep your legs extended and your head down.
3. Try to touch your toes and hold.
   Note: This stretch should be done slowly.

Sprinter Start

Stretches the groin and inner muscles of your thigh, the groin and front of the thigh, and the groin and front of the ankle, respectively.

1. Stand with your right leg forward and bend it as you lean forward, sliding your left leg back as far as possible. Keep the left leg straight. Place both hands on the floor on either side of the right foot for support.
2. Point toes (a) out to the side and hold; (b) straight and hold; (c) inward and hold.
3. Repeat for the right leg.

Single-Leg Raises

Improves the flexibility of the muscles at the back of your thighs.

1. Lie on your back with knees bent and hands by your sides.
2. Bring the right knee toward the chest, then push the right heel toward the ceiling. Keep the left leg bent.
3. Straighten your right leg and pull your toes toward the floor. Hold.
4. Repeat for the left leg.
   Note: A 90-degree angle between your straight legs and hips is desirable.

If you wish, try the following tension release exercises.

Deep Breathing

1. Lie on your back with the legs bent, feet flat on the floor, and hands by your sides.
2. Take a deep breath, hold for one to two seconds, and blow out.
3. Repeat five to six times.

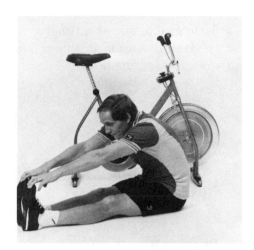

Sitting Leg Stretch

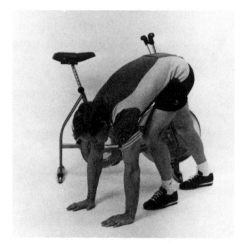

Sprinter Start

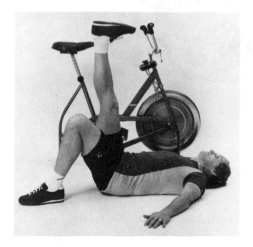

Single Leg Raises

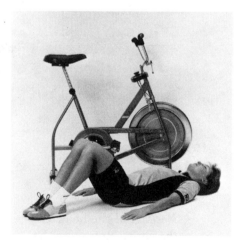

Deep Breathing

Muscle Tension and Release

1. Lie on your back, legs extended, arms at your sides.
2. Tighten the feet, lower legs, thighs, hips, stomach, low back, chest, upper back, hands, forearms, shoulders, neck, and face. Keep everything tight for three to four seconds, then release.
3. Repeat, concentrating on each muscle group, one at a time. Focus on the muscle group and release all tension in those muscles. Start with the feet and work toward the head.

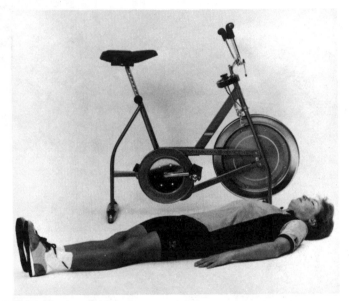

Muscle Tension and Release

Body Relaxation

All of these exercises are to be performed while lying on your back with legs bent:

- *Neck:* Roll the head all the way to the left, then all the way to the right. Return to the starting position. Take a deep breath. Release and repeat.
- *Shoulders:* Shrug the shoulders up, hold, and release. Take a deep breath. Release and repeat.
- *Arms:* While keeping the elbow on the floor, raise the right arm and let it flop back to the ground. Do the same with the left arm. Take a breath. Release and repeat.

- *Seat:* Tighten seat muscles and release. Take a deep breath. Release and repeat.
- *Legs:* Slide the right leg out straight and drag it back. Repeat with the left leg. Take a deep breath. Release and repeat.
- *Ankles:* Sit up and cross the right leg over the left. Hold the right ankle with your hands and rotate the ankle first in one direction, then in the other. Do the same with the left ankle. Lie down. Take a deep breath. Release and repeat.
- *Reverse:* Do the above exercises in reverse order.

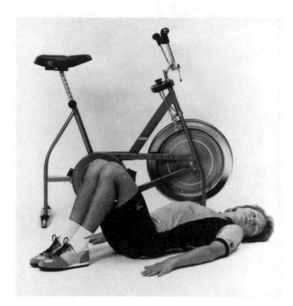

Body Relaxation

That concludes the basic training program for the exercise bike and cycle ergometer. One final word as a precautionary measure: always listen to your body when exercising. Table 10, on the following pages, summarizes complaints you may experience, the probable chief cause of each complaint, and the suggested treatment. Note that the majority of complaints are caused by exercising too vigorously. Remember, your goal is improved health, well-being, and fitness. So, as you train, follow these guidelines carefully.

Table 10:
Warning Signs, Cause, and Treatment of Overtraining

Complaint	Cause	Treatment
"My heart feels funny." (This may be a hollow feeling, a fluttering, a sudden racing, or a slowing of the heart rate.)	Your bicycling is too vigorous.	Slow down intensity of bicycling and see your doctor.
"I have a sharp pain or pressure in my chest."	Your bicycling is too vigorous.	Slow down intensity of bicycling and see your doctor.
"I am dizzy or light-headed"; "My head feels funny"; "I break out into a cold sweat"; or "I almost fainted."	Your bicycling is too vigorous. Not enough blood gets to your brain.	Slow down intensity of bicycling and see your doctor.
"My heart seems to be beating too fast 5–10 minutes after bicycling" or "I seem breathless 5–10 minutes after bicycling."	Your bicycling is too vigorous.	Work at a lower level of training heart rate range. In some instances you may need to work below that. If this doesn't correct the problem, see your doctor.
"I feel like vomiting" or "I vomit right after bicycling."	Your bicycling is too vigorous or you need a better cool-down.	Work at a lower level of training heart rate range. Take longer for a cool-down.
"I'm tired for at least a day after bicycling" or "I'm tired most of the time."	Your bicycling is too vigorous.	Work at a lower level of training heart rate range. Work to a higher level more gradually or you may need more sleep/rest.
"I can't sleep at night after bicycling."	Your bicycling is too vigorous or done too late in the evening.	Ride your bike at least 2–3 hours before retiring or ride at a lower level of training heart rate.

Complaint	Cause	Treatment
"Even though I'm bicycling, my nerves seem shot"; "I'm jittery"; or "I'm hyper all the time."	Too much bicycling or too much competition.	Lay off the competition (i.e., working against the clock), cut back on your intensity, and/or switch to another activity for a short time.
"I've lost my zing" or "I'm no longer interested in my favorite activity."	Too much bicycling or too much competition.	Lay off the competition (i.e., working against the clock), cut back on your intensity, and/or switch to another activity for a short time.
"During the first few minutes of bicycling I can't get my breath."	Improper warm-up.	Spend more time on your warm-up, at least 10 minutes, until you get to your training heart rate range.

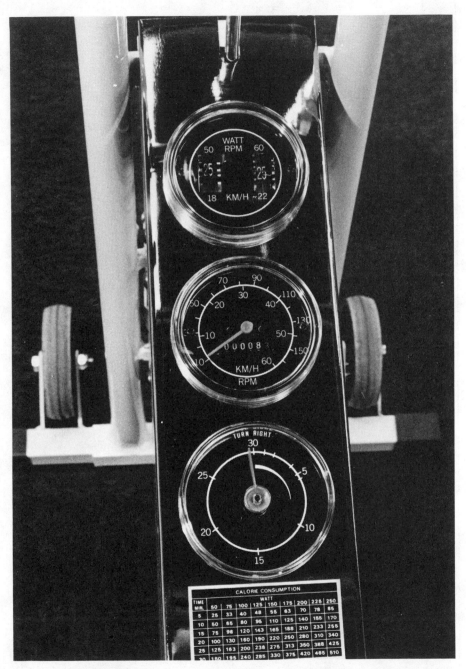

The dials and gadgets on an ergometer may look confusing, but they'll really help you to have a good workout.

5

THE CYCLE ERGOMETER

YOUR CYCLE ERGOMETER has an impressive array of dials, gadgets, and numbers. While they may be intimidating at first, they can be used to condition your body accurately and safely (see photo on page 56).

The dials, numbers, and calibrations allow you to establish or use work loads based on internationally recognized work units. These units are especially important if you're following a carefully prescribed exercise program to improve your health and performance or even rehabilitate you from a heart attack, under the direction of a physician, an exercise physiologist, or a coach.

On the following pages is a program using the various work units found on your ergometer. If you have an exercise bicycle instead of an ergometer, you may go on to Chapter 6.

The cycle ergometer can be used to measure your physical fitness and determine personal fitness programs based on calories, METS, and oxygen usage. First, let's look at how the ergometer measures your physical fitness.

THE PHYSICAL FITNESS TEST

To get the most out of your cycle ergometer, you should start with a test of your aerobic fitness. *Aerobic fitness* refers to the capacity of your body to carry oxygen to your muscle cells. The higher your oxygen-carrying capacity is, the higher your fitness level.

In a laboratory, scientists determine the amount of oxygen a person uses. At rest, it is about one-quarter to one-fifth of a liter (a liter is a little more than a quart) of oxygen a minute. During heavy, maximum exercise, it may be three to five liters a minute. A really fit athlete may use six liters a minute.

If you look closely at your cycle ergometer, you will see at least two work load measurements: watts and kilograms. These units refer or correspond to oxygen used. See Table 11 for the relationship. For example, if you work at 1,200 kpm (kilopoundmeter) or 200 watts, you are supposedly using 2.8 liters of oxygen. If your maximum work load was 300 watts or 1,800 kpm, your maximum oxygen uptake would be 4.2 liters per minute. That would be a pretty good effort and a sign of generally good aerobic fitness.

Table 11:
Work Loads and Oxygen Uptake

| Work Load | | Oxygen Uptake |
watts	kpm/min	liters/min
50	300	0.9
100	600	1.5
150	900	2.1
200	1200	2.8
250	1500	3.5
300	1800	4.2
350	2100	5.0
400	2400	5.7
450	2700	6.4

Over the years, scientists have determined that body size greatly influences oxygen usage. For example, during the same amount of exercise a big man might use five liters of oxygen per minute while a smaller man uses three liters of oxygen. Therefore, scientists prefer to express oxygen usage or uptake in relation to body weight. That way, all men and women are treated equally.

Because of the scientists' desire to keep the measurements equal, they express oxygen usage in milliliters (1,000ths of a liter) of oxygen per kilogram (2.2 pounds) of body weight per minute (ml/kg/min). With this method of measurement, it is possible to compare individuals of different sizes. Some scientists call this measurement *maximum aerobic power*, that is, your body's maximum ability to use oxygen.

As you would expect, the best-trained endurance athletes (marathon runners and cyclists) have maximum aerobic power values that far exceed the average person's value. On the average, men have maximum aerobic power scores of 35–45 ml/kg/min; women have scores of 30–40 ml/kg/min. The trained endurance athlete's score will be twice as high. The maximum aerobic power of some Olympic endurance-trained male athletes exceeds 90 ml/kg/min; female athletes' maximum exceeds 75 ml/kg/min.

Because of the adjustments that must be made for weight, the Table 11 oxygen uptake scores of a 110- or 220-pound person would be adjusted as shown in Table 12. These new scores (ml/kg/min) will allow you to determine your physical fitness (aerobic power) levels. But more on that later.

You were told earlier (Chapter 4) that there is a parallel increase in heart rate and oxygen uptake. We will take advantage of that relationship here in helping you determine your physical fitness level.

Table 12:
Work Loads and Oxygen Uptake

Work Load		Oxygen Uptake		
			ml/kg/min	
watts	kpm/min	liters/min	110 lbs.	220 lbs.
50	300	0.9	18	9
100	600	1.5	30	15
150	900	2.1	42	21
200	1200	2.8	54	27
250	1500	3.5	78	39
300	1800	4.2	82	41
350	2100	5.0	100	50
400	2400	5.7	114	57
450	2700	6.4	128	64

GETTING READY

1. The test should take place in a room that is well ventilated and comfortable (65–68° F.).
2. Do *not* eat for two hours before the test.
3. Do *not* smoke for two hours before the test.
4. Do *not* do heavy exercise for four hours before the test.
5. You should be well rested and free from infection, flu, or cold.
6. Wear shorts, T-shirt, and comfortable shoes.
7. Have your doctor's permission to take the test.

THE TEST

1. Make sure you are seated properly on the cycle ergometer (see Chapter 3). The handlebar position should allow the upper body to lean forward slightly.
2. Be certain the cycle ergometer dial is on the zero position at the start. (This is a rough form of calibration.)
3. Pedal for three minutes with the dial set at 300 kpm (1 kp or 50 watts) as a warm-up. The pedal frequency should be 100 downbeats per minute, that is, 50 downbeats for the right leg and 50 for the left leg. This is considered 50 revolutions per minute. Have someone count the cadence. The proper rhythm and cadence are very important.

MALE

Step 1

    a. Three-minute warm-up at 300 kpm—50 revolutions per minute (rpm).

    b. At end of warm-up, take pulse rate for 15 seconds. Record: _____ .

    c. If pulse rate is below 100 beats per minute (bpm), set work load for 750 kpm; if pulse rate is above 100 bpm, set work load for 600 kpm.

Step 2
- a. Cycle for three minutes at 750 kpm or 600 kpm—50 rpm. Take pulse for 15 seconds. Record: _____.
- b. If pulse rate is below 120 bpm, set work load for 1,200 kpm; if pulse rate is above 120 bpm, set work load for 1,050 kpm.

Step 3
- a. Cycle for three minutes at 1,200 kpm or 1,050 kpm—50 rpm. Take pulse for 15 seconds. Record: _____.

Go to Chart 2 on page 63 and plot your pulse rate for steps 2 and 3. Follow the directions on the chart. A sample chart, Chart 1, is shown on page 62.

FEMALE

Step 1
- a. Three-minute warm-up at 150 kpm—50 revolutions per minute (rpm).
- b. At end of warm-up, take pulse rate for 15 seconds. Record: _____.
- c. If pulse rate is below 100 beats per minute (bpm), set work load for 450 kpm; if pulse rate is above 100 bpm, set work load for 300 kpm.

Step 2
- a. Cycle for three minutes at 450 kpm or 300 kpm—50 rpm. Take pulse for 15 seconds. Record: _____.
- b. If pulse rate is below 125 bpm, set work load for 750 kpm; if pulse rate is above 125 bpm, set work load for 600 kpm.

Step 3
- a. Cycle for three minutes at 750 kpm or 600 kpm—50 rpm. Take your pulse for 15 seconds. Record: _____.

Now go to Chart 2 on page 63 and plot your pulse rates for steps 2 and 3. Follow the directions on the chart. A sample chart, Chart 1, is shown on page 62.

Chart 1:
Your Predicted Maximum Aerobic Power

(Sample)

NAME _____ AGE _____ WEIGHT _____ lbs.

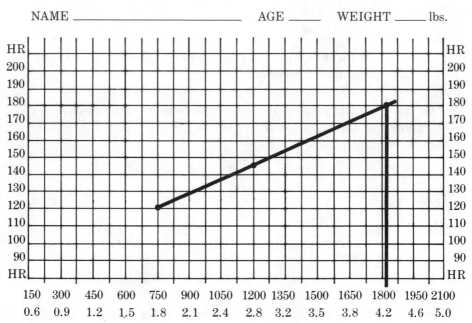

Here is an example of a 40-year-old male (maximum heart rate 180) with work load pulse rates of 120 (2a) and 145 (3a). This person has a maximum work load of slightly more than 1,800 kilograms and a maximum aerobic power of 4.2 liters.

Chart 2:
Your Predicted Maximum Aerobic Power

Directions

1. Record your pulse rates from steps 2a and 3a on pages 60–61 (males) or page 61 (females).
   Pulse rate 2a _____ and 3a _____.
2. Plot your heart rate for step 2a on the graph.
3. Plot your heart rate for step 3a on the graph.
4. Determine your maximum heart rate (220 minus age). Draw a line across your graph at your maximum heart rate.
5. Draw a line through pulse rates plotted (2a and 3a). Then extend the line to the maximum heart rate for your age.
6. Where the line intersects your maximum heart rate, drop a line to the baseline. At the baseline you will see your predicted maximum work load and oxygen uptake.

(Sample)

NAME _____ AGE _____ WEIGHT _____ lbs.

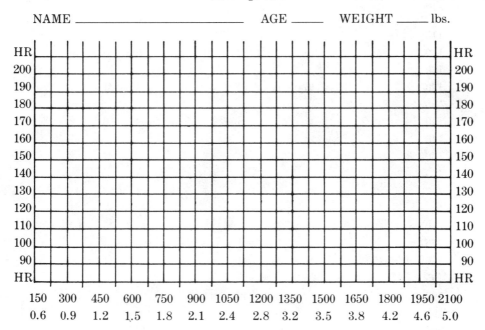

Now that you have your maximum aerobic power in liters per minute, it's time to adjust that figure to your ml/kg/min. Table 13 does that for you. Find your weight on the left, predicted maximum aerobic power at the top from Chart 2 on page 63, and read the graph mileage-map style. You now have your ml/kg score. Example: A 170-pound person with a predicted maximum aerobic power of 4.2 would have a 55 ml/kg score.

Table 13:
Calculation of Maximum Oxygen Uptake—ml/kg/min

Body Weight	Maximum Oxygen Uptake—liters per minute										
(pounds)	1.5	1.8	2.1	2.4	2.8	3.2	3.5	3.8	4.2	4.6	5.0
110	30	36	42	48	56	64	70	76	84	92	100
115											
120	28	33	39	44	52	59	65	70	78	85	93
125											
130	25	31	36	41	47	54	59	64	71	78	85
135											
140	23	28	33	38	44	50	55	59	66	72	78
145											
150	22	26	31	35	41	47	51	56	62	68	74
155											
160	21	25	29	33	38	44	48	52	58	63	68
165											
170	19	23	27	31	36	42	45	49	55	60	65
175											
180	18	22	26	29	34	39	43	46	51	56	61
185											
190	17	21	24	28	33	37	41	44	49	53	58
195											
200	16	20	23	26	31	35	38	42	46	51	55
205											
210	16	19	22	25	29	34	37	40	44	48	53
215											
220	15	18	21	24	28	32	35	38	42	46	50

Table 14:
Fitness Classification Based on ml/kg/min

Age	Very Low	Fair	Average	Good	Excellent
Women:					
20–29	28 or less	29–34	35–43	44–48	49 and above
30–39	27 or less	28–33	34–41	42–47	48 and above
40–49	25 or less	26–31	32–40	41–44	46 and above
50–59	21 or less	22–28	29–36	37–41	42 and above
Men:					
20–29	38 or less	39–43	44–51	52–56	57 and above
30–39	34 or less	35–39	40–47	48–51	52 and above
40–49	30 or less	31–35	36–43	44–47	48 and above
50–59	25 or less	26–31	32–39	40–43	44 and above
60–69	21 or less	22–26	27–35	36–39	40 and above

That's it! You now have your physical fitness score and your maximum oxygen uptake, without a lot of expense.

YOUR CYCLE ERGOMETER PROGRAM

Once you have your fitness level—and your maximum aerobic power—and your maximum work load, you can establish your personal cycle ergometer program. To get the most out of this program, work at 50–80 percent of your potential maximum effort.

Look at Table 15 on the following page. Your ergometer will use one, all, or any combination of the work units included in the table.

Recall your maximum work load from Chart 2. Now find your maximum work load on Table 15. To the immediate right of your maximum work load you'll find your training work load. To condition your body, you should work at your training work load for 30 minutes three to five times a week. Remember, if your goal is cardiovascular fitness, exercise a minimum of three times a week. If your goal is weight control, exercise a minimum of four times a week.

Table 15:
Work Units on Cycle Ergometer

Kgm	Training Work Load	Kp	Training Work Load	Watt	Training Work Load	NM	Training Work Load	Joule	Training Work Load
150	75– 120	.5	.25– .40	25	12.5– 20.0	5	2.5– 4.0	25	12.5– 20.0
300	150– 240	1.0	.50– .80	50	25.0– 40.0	10	5.0– 8.0	50	25.0– 40.0
450	225– 360	1.5	.75–1.20	75	37.5– 60.0	15	7.5–12.0	75	37.5– 60.0
600	300– 480	2.0	1.00–1.60	100	50.0– 80.0	20	10.0–16.0	100	50.0– 80.0
750	375– 600	2.5	1.25–2.00	125	62.5–100.0	25	12.5–20.0	125	62.5–100.0
900	450– 720	3.0	1.50–2.40	150	75.0–120.0	30	15.0–24.0	150	75.0–120.0
1050	525– 840	3.5	1.75–2.80	175	87.5–140.0	35	17.5–28.0	175	87.5–140.0
1200	600– 960	4.0	2.00–3.20	200	100.0–160.0	40	20.0–32.0	200	100.0–160.0
1350	675–1080	4.5	2.25–3.60	225	112.5–180.0	45	22.5–36.0	225	112.5–180.0
1500	750–1200	5.0	2.50–4.00	250	125.0–200.0	50	25.0–40.0	250	125.0–200.0
1650	825–1320	5.5	2.75–4.40	275	137.5–220.0	55	27.5–44.0	275	137.5–220.0
1800	900–1440	6.0	3.00–4.80	300	150.0–240.0	60	30.0–48.0	300	150.0–240.0
1950	975–1560	6.5	3.25–5.20	325	162.5–260.0	65	32.5–52.0	325	162.5–260.0
2100	1050–1680	7.0	3.50–5.60	350	175.0–280.0	70	35.0–56.0	350	175.0–280.0

As a check, you may want to take your heart rate when exercising. If you're riding the cycle in the training work load range recorded, I'll bet your heart rate will be between 55 and 75 percent of maximum (see Tables 2–7).

6

TRAINING FOR SPORTS

TRAINING FOR SPORT requires that you condition your body with a program that closely resembles the intensity and action of your sport. Whether your sport requires a good bit of stop-and-go action (basketball) or continuous play (soccer), your training should be oriented toward that type of play. The patterning of your training for your sport is often called *specificity of training*. *Specificity of training* means that the muscles used in your sport and the body's energy systems must be trained. The latter point is the topic of this chapter.

Your body derives its energy for muscular contraction and action from a chemical substance known as *adenosine triphosphate*, ATP for short. ATP is supplied to your muscles by three major energy systems that work independently and together to supply you with energy. The energy system in charge at any one time depends on how hard and how long you are doing the activity.

For example, if you run all-out for 10 seconds, one system predominates. If you run for an hour, a second system is in charge. As you would expect, there is also an intermediate system for those activities that last longer than 10 seconds but less than an hour.

Physiologists have given names to these systems. The system for short bursts of intense effort is called the *ATP system*. The second, or intermediate, system is called the *lactic acid system (LA system)*. The third system is called the *oxygen system (O₂ system)*.

When producing energy (ATP) for your body, the different systems are called on to assist one another. That is, one system does not suddenly stop, with the other taking over. Instead, these systems interact.

The ATP system totally predominates for the first 10 seconds of intense effort. After 30 seconds of exercise, the ATP system contributes 50 percent of the ATP and the LA system contributes the other 50 percent. Fifty seconds into exercise, the LA system contributes 75 percent of the ATP and the ATP and O_2 systems contribute the rest. Ninety seconds into the event, it's a 50-50 split between the LA and O_2 systems. And finally, at 2 minutes or more, the O_2 system is carrying 75 percent or more of the load and the LA system the rest.

Chart 3 shows the approximate contribution of each system to the replenishment of energy for the muscle, or ATP.

Chart 3

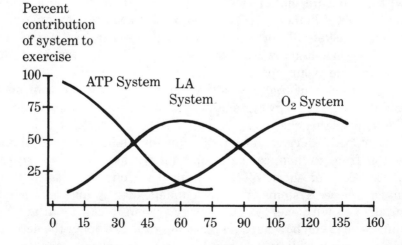

Time (in seconds) of exercise

Physiologists say that the ATP and LA systems are anaerobic. That is, they produce ATP without oxygen being present. On the other hand, the O_2 system is aerobic. It requires the presence of oxygen to produce ATP. Without enough oxygen, the muscles are capable of only a short period of work.

Let's use a couple of illustrations. At one time, your physical education teacher may have had you run 50 meters all-out. Believe it or not, you could have run the entire distance holding your breath. Afterward, you were gasping for breath, but you were able to sprint the 50 meters and meet the demands for the effort by using the ATP stored in your muscles. During this run, your ATP system was in charge.

On another occasion, you may have been told to run all-out for 400 meters—one time around the old high school track. At the start you felt good, but as you rounded the last turn, rigor mortis set in. Your arm muscles tightened, breathing was labored, leg muscles were heavy, and your running form deteriorated. You felt the proverbial "bear on your back." You experienced an excessive amount of lactic acid buildup in your bloodstream from the intense effort.

The buildup of lactic acid and the resulting fatigue occurred because you could not take in enough oxygen to meet the demands of your muscles. Your ATP was depleted.

After the run, you collapsed. You breathed deeply and heavily and in time replaced your body with oxygen, and your ATP was restored. You were ready to run another 400 meters (only if your life depended on it). During the 400-meter run, your LA system was in charge. Of course, your ATP and O_2 systems assisted.

Last, but not least, you were asked to run 1½ miles as fast as possible. (These phys ed teachers sure were gluttons for punishment—your punishment.) In the mile-and-a-half run, a new energy system was used—your oxygen or aerobic system. You probably remember from your high school biology days that no one can survive long without oxygen. After a few minutes without oxygen, there will be no ATP. No ATP means no energy; no energy means the cells die; cell death results in bodily death.

With adequate amounts of oxygen, the foods you eat (fats or carbohydrates—sugar, starches) provide you with a constant supply of ATP to be used by your muscle cells. So, when you ran 1½ miles nonstop you ran at a pace that allowed you to take in enough oxygen to meet the demands of your muscles.

Of course, near the end of the run you gave it the old high school try (you wanted an A in phys ed). You quickened your pace on the last lap. You pushed yourself to your limits, and the LA and ATP systems came into play. The 1½-mile run went from a pay-as-you-go activity to an all-out sprint such as the 400-meter run.

Got it? To make sure, let's capsulize the energy systems. That way, you'll understand how and why sport training systems are set up.

ANAEROBIC—WITHOUT OXYGEN

1. The ATP System. The immediate demand for ATP is supplied to the muscles by this system. It taps the stored ATP in the muscles for immediate use. ATP is replenished by a breakdown of another chemical called *phosphocreatine*—PC for short. Because of this, physiologists prefer to call the ATP system the *ATP-PC system*. Although this system supplies energy quickly, the limited supply of ATP is exhausted after 8–10 seconds of all-out effort.

2. The LA System. This system provides ATP rapidly. It produces ATP in a process that involves the incomplete breakdown of carbohydrates. The LA system provides energy for all-out efforts that last from 30 seconds to 3 minutes. The LA system also is responsible for producing lactic acid. When the level of lactic acid gets too high, fatigue occurs and physical activity must stop.

AEROBIC

3. The O_2 System. This system supplies you with a great deal of ATP. If you are in good physical condition and exercise on a pay-as-you-go basis (walking, leisurely bicycling, jogging), you can breathe deeply enough so you can take in enough oxygen to supply you with adequate levels of ATP.

INTERACTION AMONG THE THREE SYSTEMS

Many times in exercising, there is a strong interplay between the LA and O_2 systems. During an all-out 5K (3.1-mile) run, you will be pushing yourself beyond your oxygen limits and going to what is called your *anaerobic threshold*.

When you are jogging or running easily, your demand for

oxygen is supplied constantly. This is called *steady-state exercise.* But, when you quicken your pace at the end of a race and push yourself to beat an opponent, your body's demand for oxygen can no longer be met. So, your anaerobic (ATP and LA) systems kick in. Lactic acid is produced. This is your anaerobic threshold. Your anaerobic threshold is reached at about 90 percent of your maximum effort. A well-trained athlete conditions his or her body so that the anaerobic threshold is pushed back, and the athlete can push longer and harder. By raising the anaerobic threshold (best done through interval training), the athlete can start the sprint or kick to the finish earlier and at an even greater intensity. Between evenly matched athletes, the victory usually goes to the athlete with the higher anaerobic threshold.

If all this biochemistry fries your brain, just remember the following:

1. Your body uses three different energy systems to replenish ATP.
2. There is an overlap among the three systems.
3. The energy systems must be trained near their maximum (90 percent or above) to reach top sport performance levels.

IMPROVING YOUR ANAEROBIC THRESHOLD AND SPORT PERFORMANCE THROUGH INTERVAL TRAINING

Because of the overlap of the three energy systems and the need to stimulate them near their maximum, physiologists have determined that there are *four* training efforts, as follows.

Training Effort I (ATP System). These are training activities that are short bursts of incredible effort (90–95 percent of maximum). They take 30 seconds or less. Sprint cycling, 50-meter runs, tennis serves, and power weightlifting fall into this category. This is called an *anaerobic activity.*

Training Effort II (ATP and LA Systems). These are activities that last from 30 seconds to 1½ minutes. The kilometer in cycling, 200- to 400-meter runs, speed skating, and 100-yard swims fall into this category. This, too, is an anaerobic activity.

Training Effort III (LA and O$_2$ Systems). These are activities that last 1½–3 minutes. The 800-meter dash, floor gymnastics, and wrestling all fall into this category. These activities are primarily anaerobic with some aerobic (with oxygen) emphasis.

Training Effort IV (O₂ System). These are activities that last longer than three minutes. Two-mile runs, lacrosse games, cross-country skiing, and most outdoor cycling activities fall into this aerobic area.

As you would expect, no one sport really focuses on one energy system or one training effort. Sprinters run more than one race and need proper conditioning to make repeat efforts in practice and at athletic events. Marathon runners and cyclists primarily use the O₂ system, but they also push themselves near the end of the race or with surges during the race. So the training efforts and energy systems are best combined for optimum sport performance. Training plans usually combine the various efforts as follows:

Plan 1. Combine the ATP and LA systems in training for sports that require relatively short bursts of effort, taking from a few seconds to 1½ minutes. Sprinting in running, swimming, and cycling are perfect examples.

Plan 2. Combine the ATP, LA, and O₂ systems for sports that last 1½–3 minutes (800- to 1,000-meter runs in track). The kilometer in cycling, wrestling, and boxing are best suited to this type of training.

Plan 3. The LA and O₂ systems should be combined for sports that last for three minutes or longer but do require intense efforts at times. Soccer, lacrosse, field hockey, road racing in running, and distance cycling fall into this category.

These training efforts and combinations must be remembered when designing your sport training system.

Your sport training is best accomplished through interval training. Interval training is a series of repeated bouts of hard exercise alternated with periods of rest. Light exercise usually constitutes the rest period.

Before reading about plans for interval training, you should understand one concept. Interval training allows you to do more work than other forms of training. Let me explain: Suppose you rode a bicycle as hard as possible for 1 minute. At the end, you would be exhausted. But now suppose you rode intermittently. That is, you rode just as hard for 10 seconds as you did for 1 minute, then rested 30 seconds, then rode again for 10 seconds. If you followed this pattern of 10 seconds of hard riding and 30 seconds of rest 6 times, you would perform the same amount of work as 1 minute (6 bouts × 10 seconds = 60 seconds). There would, however, be one difference. You would have felt much less fatigue after the interval training than after the continuous training. If you doubt it, try it sometime and see for yourself.

The reason for the difference is that hard training with intermittent rest means less lactic acid buildup and less fatigue. Lactic acid, as you recall, slows production of ATP. The key is rest. The rest allows you to breathe in enough oxygen to reduce the buildup of lactic acid and continue training for longer periods of time at high intensities.

The bottom line in all of this is that with interval training you will be able to train longer and harder (push back the anaerobic threshold) than with continuous training.

As you would expect, the longer the rest period, the greater the amount of ATP that is restored. According to the late Dr. Ed Fox, the following rest intervals produce these percentages of ATP restored (Table 16).

Table 16:
Rest Periods and Percentage of ATP Restored

Rest Period	Percentage of ATP System Restored
Less than 10 seconds	Minimal
30 seconds	50%
60 seconds	75%
90 seconds	88%
120 seconds	94%
More than 120 seconds	100%

In addition, research shows that the stroke volume of the heart (the amount of blood pumped by the heart with each beat or stroke) is highest during the *recovery* period from exercise. The higher the maximum stroke volume, the more blood and oxygen that is pumped to the exercising muscles—so aerobic power (cardiovascular fitness) is increased.

In short, interval training allows you to train harder and longer and improve your cardiovascular fitness level more than does continuous training. Because interval training is so intense, doing it daily for half a year can lead to burnout. Also, interval training should not be used for improvement of physical fitness. Instead it is to be used for conditioning and training. Every other day for eight or nine weeks is best.

Basically, interval training is patterned on a series of sets of intense efforts followed by recovery. The training pattern looks something like this:

Set 1

 Cycle hard for 20 seconds
 Rest for 60 seconds
 Cycle hard for 20 seconds
 Rest for 60 seconds
 Cycle hard for 20 seconds
 Rest for 60 seconds
 Cycle hard for 20 seconds
 Rest for 60 seconds
 Cycle hard for 20 seconds
 Rest 120 seconds

Set 2

 Cycle hard for 20 seconds
 Rest for 60 seconds
 Cycle hard for 20 seconds
 Rest for 60 seconds
 Cycle hard for 20 seconds
 Rest for 60 seconds
 Cycle hard for 20 seconds
 Rest for 60 seconds
 Cycle hard for 20 seconds
 Rest 120 seconds

Set 3

 Cycle hard for 20 seconds
 Rest for 60 seconds
 Cycle hard for 20 seconds
 Rest for 60 seconds
 Cycle hard for 20 seconds
 Rest for 60 seconds
 Cycle hard for 20 seconds
 Rest for 60 seconds

Cycle hard for 20 seconds
Rest 120 seconds
To save space, this training pattern would be written as:

Set 1: 5 × 0:20 (rest 1:00)
Rest 2:00
Set 2: 5 × 0:20 (rest 1:00)
Rest 2:00
Set 3: 5 × 0:20 (rest 1:00)

Now that you understand how interval training programs are set up, it's time to understand how to use your pulse rate in interval training.

As with continuous aerobic training (Chapter 4), your pulse rate can be used to estimate your optimum exercise for interval training. Your pulse rate will tell you your peak or training heart rate during exercise. That will be somewhere between 85 and 95 percent of your maximum heart rate, depending on your age and type of training.

Your pulse rate will also be used to indicate when you have recovered sufficiently from the hard exercise to go at it again.

To be perfectly honest, you can use the interval training programs without your pulse rate—you push yourself to near exhaustion for the specific period of time—and then rest for the time allotted. The pulse rate, however, allows you to be a bit more scientific and more accurate.

Table 17, on the following page, is a summary of your training and recovery heart rates. The training heart rates were established by taking 85–95 percent of your assumed maximum heart rate (Table 1) (I–III, 85–95 percent; III and IV, 85–90 percent). The recovery rates were determined by taking 75 and 62.5 percent, respectively, of your assumed maximum heart rate (Table 1) (I by 75 percent; II by 62.5 percent). Look at Table 17 to determine your personal training heart rate and recovery rate. A 20-year-old, for example, would train at the following heart rates:

Cycle efforts under 1.5 minutes: 186–200 bpm
Cycle efforts 1.5–3 minutes: 166–190 bpm
Cycle efforts over 3 minutes: 166–180 bpm

The recovery heart rate would be 147–150 bpm between repetitions and 123–125 between sets.

Table 17:
Specific Training and Recovery Heart Rates
Suggested for Interval Training

	Training Heart Rates		Recovery Heart Rates	
	Training Efforts	Training Efforts		
AGE	Less than 3 minutes (85–95% of max)	3 minutes or more (85–90% of max)	Repetitions	Sets
15–19	171–195	171–185	151–154	126–128
20–24	166–190	166–180	147–150	123–125
25–29	161–185	161–175	143–146	120–122
30–34	156–180	156–170	139–142	113–119
35–39	151–175	151–165	136–138	113–116
40–44	146–170	146–160	132–135	110–112
45–49	141–165	141–155	128–131	107–109
50–54	136–160	136–150	124–127	104–106
55–59	131–155	131–145	120–123	100–103
60 +	Not recommended			

With all of that theory as background, it's time to provide three possible interval training programs for various sports. With these programs, keep in mind that, if the training effort calls for efforts of less than three minutes, your heart rate is to be at 85-95 percent of maximum. If it is three minutes or more, your heart rate is to be at 85-90 percent of maximum (see Table 17). Your rest periods between repetitions and sets are also found in Table 17.

The following training plans, in Tables 18, 19, and 20, permit you to use indoor cycling as a means of training for your favorite sport. For sports in Category A, during the first day of the first week you will cycle at 90-95 percent of your maximum effort for 20 seconds and finish with easy cycling during the rest phase.

Sports Category A includes archery, bowling, cycling (1,000m-1Km), discus, golf, javelin, running (100-200m), shot put, boxing, fencing, football, gymnastics, judo, karate, wrestling, basketball, volleyball, baseball, hockey, lacrosse, and soccer. Category B includes running (400m), downhill skiing, swimming (400m), badminton, handball, racquetball, squash, and tennis. Category C includes running or cross-country skiing (1-6mi), marathons, and distance cycling.

Table 18:
Interval Training for Sports in Category A

Training Plans for Sports in Category A
Weeks/Days

First Week		Fourth Week	
1	8 x 0:20 (rest 1:00)	1	4 x 3:00 (rest 3:00)
2	2 x 2:00 (rest 4:00) Rest 2:00 1 x 2:00 (rest 4:00)	2	4 x 0:40 (rest 1:55) Rest 2:00 8 x 0:20 (rest 0:55) Rest 2:00 8 x 0:20 (rest 0:55)
3	8 x 0:20 (rest 1:00) Rest 2:00 8 x 0:20 (rest 1:00)	3	4 x 2:00 (rest 2:00)
Second Week		**Fifth Week**	
1	3 x 2:00 (rest 4:00) Rest 2:00 2 x 2:00 (rest 4:00)	1	4 x 0:40 (rest 1:50) Rest 2:00 8 x 0:20 (rest 0:45) Rest 2:00 8 x 0:20 (rest 0:45)
2	4 x 0:40 (rest 2:00) Rest 2:00 8 x 0:20 (rest 1:00) Rest 2:00 8 x 0:20 (rest 1:00)	2	5 x 2:00 (rest 4:00)
3	4 x 3:00 (rest 3:00)	3	4 x 0:40 (rest 1:50) Rest 2:00 8 x 0:20 (rest 0:45) Rest 2:00 8 x 0:20 (rest 0:45)
Third Week			
1	4 x 0:40 (rest 2:00) Rest 2:00 8 x 0:20 (rest 2:00) Rest 2:00 8 x 0:20 (rest 2:00)	**Sixth Week**	
		1	4 x 0:40 (rest 1:50) Rest 2:00 8 x 0:20 (rest 0:45) Rest 2:00 8 x 0:20 (rest 0:45)
2	4 x 3:00 (rest 3:00)	2	3 x 3:30 (rest 3:30)
3	4 x 0:40 (rest 2:00) Rest 2:00 8 x 0:20 (rest 2:00) Rest 2:00 8 x 0:20 (rest 2:00)	3	4 x 0:40 (rest 1:50) Rest 2:00 8 x 0:20 (rest 0:45) Rest 2:00 8 x 0:20 (rest 0:45)

(Table continued on next page.)

Table 18: cont.
Interval Training for Sports in Category A

Training Plans for Sports in Category A
Weeks/Days

Seventh Week		Ninth Week	
1	4 x 0:40 (rest 1:50) Rest 2:00 8 x 0:20 (rest 0:45) Rest 2:00 8 x 0:20 (rest 0:45)	1	4 x 0:40 (rest 1:50) Rest 2:00 3 x 4:30 (rest 2:15) Rest 2:00 8 x 0:20 (rest 0:45)
2	3 x 3:30 (rest 3:30)	2	3 x 3:30 (rest 3:30)
3	4 x 0:40 (rest 1:50) Rest 2:00 8 x 0:20 (rest 0:45) Rest 2:00 8 x 0:20 (rest 0:45)	3	4 x 0:40 (rest 1:50) Rest 2:00 3 x 4:30 (rest 2:15) Rest 2:00 8 x 0:20 (rest 0:45)
Eighth Week			
1	4 x 0:40 (rest 1:50) Rest 2:00 8 x 0:20 (rest 0:45) Rest 2:00 8 x 0:20 (rest 0:45)		
2	3 x 3:30 (rest 3:30)		
3	4 x 0:40 (rest 1:50) Rest 2:00 8 x 0:20 (rest 0:45) Rest 2:00 8 x 0:20 (rest 0:45)		

Table 19:
Interval Training for Sports in Category B

Training Plans for Sports in Category B
Weeks/Days

First Week		Fourth Week	
1	8 x 0:20 (rest 1:00)	1	4 x 3:00 (rest 3:00)
2	2 x 2:00 (rest 4:00)	2	4 x 0:40 (rest 1:55)
	Rest 2:00		Rest 2:00
	1 x 2:00 (rest 4:00)		8 x 0:20 (rest 0:55)
3	8 x 0:20 (rest 1:00)		Rest 2:00
	Rest 2:00		8 x 0:20 (rest 0:55)
	8 x 0:20 (rest 1:00)	3	4 x 2:00 (rest 2:00)
Second Week		**Fifth Week**	
1	3 x 2:00 (rest 4:00)	1	4 x 0:40 (rest 1:50)
	Rest 2:00		Rest 2:00
	2 x 2:00 (rest 4:00)		8 x 0:20 (rest 0:45)
2	4 x 0:40 (rest 2:00)		Rest 2:00
	Rest 2:00		8 x 0:20 (rest 0:45)
	8 x 0:20 (rest 1:00)	2	5 x 2:00 (rest 4:00)
	Rest 2:00	3	4 x 0:40 (rest 1:50)
	8 x 0:20 (rest 1:00)		Rest 2:00
3	4 x 3:00 (rest 3:00)		8 x 0:20 (rest 0:45)
Third Week			Rest 2:00
1	4 x 2:00 (rest 4:00)		8 x 0:20 (rest 0:45)
	Rest 2:00	**Sixth Week**	
	2 x 1:20 (rest 2:40)	1	2 x 3:00 (rest 3:00)
2	4 x 0:40 (rest 2:00)		Rest 2:00
	Rest 2:00		2 x 1:30 (rest 3:00)
	4 x 0:40 (rest 2:00)	2	4 x 0:40 (rest 1:50)
	Rest 2:00		Rest 2:00
	4 x 0:40 (rest 2:00)		4 x 0:40 (rest 1:50)
	Rest 2:00		Rest 2:00
	4 x 0:40 (rest 2:00)		4 x 0:40 (rest 1:50)
3	2 x 3:00 (rest 3:00)		Rest 2:00
	Rest 2:00		4 x 0:40 (rest 1:50)
	2 x 1:20 (rest 2:40)	3	1 x 4:30 (rest 2:15)
			2 x 3:30 (rest 1:45)

(Table continued on next page.)

Table 19: cont.
Interval Training for Sports in Category B

Training Plans for Sports in Category B
Weeks/Days

Seventh Week		Ninth Week	
1	4 x 0:40 (rest 1:50)	1	2 x 3:00 (rest 3:00)
	Rest 2:00		Rest 2:00
	8 x 0:20 (rest 0:45)		2 x 1:30 (rest 3:00)
	Rest 2:00	2	4 x 0:40 (rest 1:50)
	8 x 0:20 (rest 0:45)		Rest 2:00
2	3 x 3:30 (rest 3:30)		4 x 0:40 (rest 1:50)
3	4 x 0:40 (rest 1:50)		Rest 2:00
	Rest 2:00		4 x 0:40 (rest 1:50)
	8 x 0:20 (rest 0:45)		Rest 2:00
	Rest 2:00		4 x 0:40 (rest 1:50)
	8 x 0:20 (rest 0:45)	3	2 x 5:00 (rest 2:30)
			Rest 2:00
Eighth Week			3 x 1:30 (rest 3:00)
1	4 x 0:40 (rest 1:50)		
	Rest 2:00		
	8 x 0:20 (rest 0:45)		
	Rest 2:00		
	8 x 0:20 (rest 0:45)		
2	3 x 3:30 (rest 3:30)		
3	4 x 0:40 (rest 1:50)		
	Rest 2:00		
	8 x 0:20 (rest 0:45)		
	Rest 2:00		
	8 x 0:20 (rest 0:45)		

Table 20:
Interval Training for Sports in Category C

Training Plans for Sports in Category C
Weeks/Days

First Week		Third Week	
1	2 x 2:15 (rest 4:30) Rest 2:00 2 x 1:20 (rest 2:40) Rest 2:00	1	4 x 2:00 (rest 4:00) Rest 2:00 2 x 1:20 (rest 2:40)
2	4 x 0:40 (rest 2:00) Rest 2:00 4 x 0:40 (rest 2:00) Rest 2:00 4 x 0:40 (rest 2:00)	2	4 x 0:40 (rest 2:00) Rest 2:00 4 x 0:40 (rest 2:00) Rest 2:00 4 x 0:40 (rest 2:00) Rest 2:00 4 x 0:40 (rest 2:00)
3	1 x 3:00 (rest 3:00) Rest 2:00 2 x 1:20 (rest 2:40) Rest 2:00	3	2 x 3:00 (rest 3:00) Rest 2:00 2 x 1:20 (rest 2:40)
Second Week		**Fourth Week**	
1	3 x 2:10 (rest 4:20) Rest 2:00 3 x 1:20 (rest 2:40)	1	4 x 2:00 (rest 4:00) Rest 2:00 2 x 1:20 (rest 2:40)
2	4 x 0:40 (rest 2:00) Rest 2:00 4 x 0:40 (rest 2:00) Rest 2:00 4 x 0:40 (rest 2:00) Rest 2:00 4 x 0:40 (rest 2:00)	2	4 x 0:40 (rest 1:55) Rest 2:00 4 x 0:40 (rest 1:55) Rest 2:00 4 x 0:40 (rest 1:55) Rest 2:00 4 x 0:40 (rest 1:55)
3	2 x 3:00 (rest 3:00) Rest 2:00 2 x 1:20 (rest 2:40)	3	2 x 3:00 (rest 3:00) Rest 2:00 2 x 1:30 (rest 3:00)

(Table continued on next page.)

Table 20: cont.
Interval Training for Sports in Category C

	Training Plans for Sports in Category C
Weeks/Days	

Fifth Week		**Seventh Week**	
1	2 x 3:00 (rest 3:00) Rest 2:00 2 x 1:30 (rest 3:00)	1	2 x 3:00 (rest 3:00) Rest 2:00 2 x 1:30 (rest 3:00)
2	4 x 0:40 (rest 1:50) Rest 2:00 4 x 0:40 (rest 1:50) Rest 2:00 4 x 0:40 (rest 1:50) Rest 2:00 4 x 0:40 (rest 1:50)	2	4 x 0:40 (rest 1:50) Rest 2:00 4 x 0:40 (rest 1:50) Rest 2:00 4 x 0:40 (rest 1:50) Rest 2:00 4 x 0:40 (rest 1:50)
3	1 x 4:30 (rest 2:15) Rest 2:00 2 x 4:00 (rest 2:00)	3	2 x 5:00 (rest 2:30) Rest 2:00
Sixth Week		**Eighth Week**	
		1	2 x 3:00 (rest 3:00) Rest 2:00 2 x 1:30 (rest 3:00)
1	2 x 3:00 (rest 3:00) Rest 2:00 2 x 1:30 (rest 3:00)		
2	4 x 0:40 (rest 1:50) Rest 2:00 4 x 0:40 (rest 1:50) Rest 2:00 4 x 0:40 (rest 1:50) Rest 2:00 4 x 0:40 (rest 1:50)	2	4 x 0:40 (rest 1:50) Rest 2:00 4 x 0:40 (rest 1:50) Rest 2:00 4 x 0:40 (rest 1:50) Rest 2:00 4 x 0:40 (rest 1:50)
3	1 x 4:30 (rest 2:15) 2 x 3:30 (rest 1:45)	3	2 x 3:00 (rest 3:00) Rest 2:00 3 x 1:30 (rest 3:00)

(Table continued on next page.)

Table 20: cont.
Interval Training for Sports in Category C

Training Plans for Sports in Category C

Weeks/Days

Ninth Week

1
2 x 3:00 (rest 3:00)
Rest 2:00
2 x 1:30 (rest 3:00)

2
4 x 0:40 (rest 1:50)
Rest 2:00
4 x 0:40 (rest 1:50)
Rest 2:00
4 x 0:40 (rest 1:50)
Rest 2:00
4 x 0:40 (rest 1:50)

3
2 x 5:00 (rest 2:30)
Rest 2:00
3 x 1:30 (rest 3:00)

One more point: Athletes report, and researchers support the observation, that athletes are better able to tolerate the intensity of interval training if they have spent about six months training aerobically. That is, before the interval training begins, they spend six months running, biking, or swimming—doing what is called, obviously, *Long Slow Distance* or *Long Steady Distance*. This training provides the athletes with a base of training. With this base, they can do the required efforts of interval work and recover more quickly during the rest periods.

Your training schedule for your sport should look like this:

1. Season ends
2. Six months of aerobic training
3. Ten weeks of interval training on the bike prior to the start of the season
4. Season begins

7

WORKOUTS FOR SPECIAL PROBLEMS

ALL OF THE training procedures outlined so far can be followed by individuals in normal good health. Modification must be made, however, for people who have unique health situations. These include people with arthritis, asthma, emphysema, heart disease, high blood pressure, and obesity.

Each of these conditions is different and merits attention. In this chapter, programs are provided and recommendations made for individuals with these ailments (without complications). No discussion of the actual ailment is included here. As for any exercise program, it is recommended that you check with your doctor before training. Take this book along and show it to your physician. With all of these special conditions, you and your doctor will need to determine the pedaling rate—most will be 90–100 rpm—and a resistance that elicits a training heart rate.

ARTHRITIS

An exercise bicycle is good for the arthritic. Your weight is supported with the seat, and the major joints of the body—hips, knees and ankles, and back—are not subjected to the jarring that you might experience when running or walking. Do not cycle on days when the arthritis pain is acute—unless you have noticed that exercise reduces the pain. *Remember always to cycle pain-free.* Don't worry about your rate of cycling. Follow the guidelines established in Chapter 4 for the warm-up and cool-down. Your peak period, however, must be modified. It should look something like this:

- *Level 1*—Cycle for 5 minutes, 4 to 5 times a week, at a rate that feels comfortable to you. Be sure you are pain-free during the exercise.
- *Level 2*—Cycle for 10 minutes, 4 to 5 times a week, at a rate that feels comfortable to you. Be sure you are pain-free during the exercise.
- *Level 3*—Cycle for 12 minutes, 4 to 5 times a week, at a rate that feels comfortable to you. Be sure you are pain-free during the exercise.
- *Level 4*—Cycle for 15 minutes, 4 to 5 times a week, at a rate that feels comfortable to you. Be sure you are pain-free during the exercise.
- *Level 5*—Cycle for 17 minutes, 4 to 5 times a week, at a rate that feels comfortable to you. Be sure you are pain-free during the exercise.
- *Level 6*—Cycle for 20 minutes, 4 to 5 times a week, at a rate that feels comfortable to you. Be sure you are pain-free during the exercise.
- *Level 7*—Cycle for 22 minutes, 4 to 5 times a week, at a rate that feels comfortable to you. Be sure you are pain-free during the exercise.
- *Level 8*—Cycle for 25 minutes, 4 to 5 times a week, at a rate that feels comfortable to you. Be sure you are pain-free during the exercise.
- *Level 9*—Cycle for 27 minutes, 4 to 5 times a week, at a rate that feels comfortable to you. Be sure you are pain-free during the exercise.
- *Level 10*—Cycle for 30 minutes, 4 to 5 times a week, at a rate that feels comfortable to you. Be sure you are pain-free during the exercise.

Spend a minimum of one week at each level. Do not move to the next level until you feel ready for it.

You are now ready to attempt the 10-minute cycle and checking of your pulse rate as described on pages 28–31. I would suggest you keep your pulse rate below 65 percent of your maximum rate.

ASTHMA

Asthmatics seem to benefit the most from training regimens that are not continuous. For them, interval training is best. Asthmatics should not, however, work at the high intensities recorded in Chapter 6. Instead, they should work at heart rates between 40 and 75 percent of their maximum heart rate range, described in Chapter 4. Instead of riding continuously, they should cycle with periods of rest.

Their cycling pattern, after a proper warm-up, will look like this:

- *Level 1*—Cycle for 1 minute at 40–60 percent of your maximum heart rate. This is to be followed by a 1-minute rest. Repeat this cycle 5 times.
- *Level 2*—Cycle for 2 minutes at 40–60 percent of your maximum heart rate. This is to be followed by a 1-minute rest. Repeat this cycle 5 times.
- *Level 3*—Cycle for 2 minutes at 40–60 percent of your maximum heart rate. This is to be followed by a 1-minute rest. Repeat this cycle 7 times.
- *Level 4*—Cycle for 2 minutes at 40–60 percent of your maximum heart rate. This is to be followed by a 1-minute rest. Repeat this cycle 9 times.
- *Level 5*—Cycle for 2 minutes at 40–60 percent of your maximum heart rate. This is to be followed by a 1-minute rest. Repeat this cycle 11 times.
- *Level 6*—Cycle for 2 minutes at 40–60 percent of your maximum heart rate. This is to be followed by a 1-minute rest. Repeat this cycle 13 times.
- *Level 7*—Cycle for 2 minutes at 40–60 percent of your maximum heart rate. This is to be followed by a 1-minute rest. Repeat this cycle 15 times.

Spend a minimum of one week at each level. Do not move to the next level until you feel ready for it.

Once Level 7 is achieved, you can take one of the following approaches:

A. Increase your heart rate—that is, pedal for two minutes with one minute of rest 15 times. Only now provide greater resistance or pedal at a faster rate. Your heart rate should be in the 60- to 75-percent range.

OR

B. Attempt to increase the number of minutes you exercise from 2 to 2.5 minutes. If you can cycle for 2½ minutes during each exercise bout, then reduce the number of repeat cycles to 12. Each week or so, gradually increase the length of cycling by 30 seconds.

3 minutes of exercise, 1 minute of rest—10 cycles
3.5 minutes of exercise, 1 minute of rest—9 cycles
4 minutes of exercise, 1 minute of rest—8 cycles
4.5 minutes of exercise, 1 minute of rest—7 cycles
5 minutes of exercise, 1 minute of rest—6 cycles
6 minutes of exercise, 1 minute of rest—5 cycles
7 minutes of exercise, 1 minute of rest—4 cycles
8 minutes of exercise, 1 minute of rest—4 cycles
9 minutes of exercise, 1 minute of rest—3 cycles
10 minutes of exercise, 1 minute of rest—3 cycles

Continuous exercise seems to precipitate bronchospasms among asthmatics. So you must use your own body as a guide. When you determine the length of exercise that is right for you, stay at that level and increase the resistance or pedal speed and work to a heart rate of 60–75 percent.

EMPHYSEMA

Your doctor and you must determine how much exercise you can safely do. He or she should tell you your training heart rate level. Once you know that, follow these guidelines:

- *Level 1*—Cycle 1 minute, rest 1 minute, cycle 1 minute, rest 1 minute, cycle 1 minute, rest 1 minute, cycle 1 minute. Do this 3 times a week.
- *Level 2*—Cycle 1 minute, rest 1 minute, cycle 3 minutes, rest

1 minute, cycle 3 minutes, rest 1 minute, cycle 1 minute. Do this 3 times a week.

- *Level 3*—Cycle 1 minute, rest 1 minute, cycle 5 minutes, rest 1 minute, cycle 5 minutes, rest 1 minute, cycle 1 minute. Do this 3 times a week.
- *Level 4*—Cycle 1 minute, rest 1 minute, cycle 7 minutes, rest 1 minute, cycle 7 minutes, rest 1 minute, cycle 1 minute. Do this 3 times a week.
- *Level 5*—Cycle 1 minute, rest 1 minute, cycle 8 minutes, rest 1 minute, cycle 8 minutes, rest 1 minute, cycle 1 minute. Do this 3 times a week.
- *Level 6*—Cycle 1 minute, rest 1 minute, cycle 9 minutes, rest 1 minute, cycle 9 minutes, rest 1 minute, cycle 1 minute. Do this 3 times a week.
- *Level 7*—Cycle 1 minute, rest 1 minute, cycle 10 minutes, rest 1 minute, cycle 10 minutes, rest 1 minute, cycle 1 minute. Do this 3 times a week.
- *Level 8*—Cycle 1 minute, rest 1 minute, cycle 11 minutes, rest 1 minute, cycle 11 minutes, rest 1 minute, cycle 1 minute. Do this 3 times a week.
- *Level 9*—Cycle 1 minute, rest 1 minute, cycle 12 minutes, rest 1 minute, cycle 12 minutes, rest 1 minute, cycle 1 minute. Do this 3 times a week.
- *Level 10*—Cycle 1 minute, rest 1 minute, cycle 14 minutes, rest 1 minute, cycle 14 minutes, rest 1 minute, cycle 1 minute. Do this 3 times a week.
- *Level 11*—Cycle 1 minute, rest 1 minute, cycle 16 minutes, rest 1 minute, cycle 16 minutes, rest 1 minute, cycle 1 minute. Do this 3 times a week.
- *Level 12*—Cycle 1 minute, rest 1 minute, cycle 18 minutes, rest 1 minute, cycle 18 minutes, rest 1 minute, cycle 1 minute. Do this 3 times a week.
- *Level 13*—Cycle 1 minute, rest 1 minute, cycle 20 minutes, rest 1 minute, cycle 20 minutes, rest 1 minute, cycle 1 minute. Do this 3 times a week.

HEART ATTACK/HEART DISEASE

Following is a cycle exercise program you can follow if you have had a heart attack and you have your doctor's permission to exercise. This program assures you a normal and uncomplicated recovery. It also assumes that you don't need medication for relief of pain and prevention of heart irregularities. Your physician must establish your training heart rate. This will be done via a stress test. The test will indicate how high your heart rate may safely go.

- *Level 1*—Cycle 3-5 minutes, 3 times a week.
- *Level 2*—Cycle 6-8 minutes, 3 times a week.
- *Level 3*—Cycle 9-11 minutes, 3 times a week.
- *Level 4*—Cycle 12-14 minutes, 4 times a week.
- *Level 5*—Cycle 15-17 minutes, 4 times a week.
- *Level 6*—Cycle 18-20 minutes, 4 times a week.
- *Level 7*—Cycle 21-23 minutes, 4 times a week.
- *Level 8*—Cycle 24-26 minutes, 4 times a week.
- *Level 9*—Cycle 27-29 minutes, 4 times a week.
- *Level 10*—Cycle 30-32 minutes, 4 times a week.
- *Level 11*—Cycle 33-35 minutes, 4 times a week.
- *Level 12*—Cycle 36-38 minutes, 4 times a week.
- *Level 13*—Cycle 39-41 minutes, 4 times a week.
- *Level 14*—Cycle 42-44 minutes, 4 times a week.
- *Level 15*—Cycle 45-47 minutes, 4 times a week.
- *Level 16*—Cycle 48-50 minutes, 4 times a week.
- *Level 17*—Cycle 51-53 minutes, 4 times a week.
- *Level 18*—Cycle 54-56 minutes, 4 times a week.
- *Level 19*—Cycle 57-59 minutes, 4 times a week.
- *Level 20*—Cycle 60 minutes, 4 times a week.

If you need medication to manage your disease, the following plan should be followed. The physician must establish your training heart rate. This will be done via a stress test. This program should also be supervised by your doctor.

- *Level 1*—Cycle 1 minute, rest 1 minute, cycle 1 minute, rest 1 minute, cycle 1 minute, rest 1 minute, cycle 1 minute. Do this 3 times a week.
- *Level 2*—Cycle 1 minute, rest 1 minute, cycle 3 minutes, rest 1 minute, cycle 3 minutes, rest 1 minute, cycle 1 minute. Do this 3 times a week.
- *Level 3*—Cycle 1 minute, rest 1 minute, cycle 5 minutes, rest 1 minute, cycle 5 minutes, rest 1 minute, cycle 1 minute. Do this 3 times a week.

- *Level 4*—Cycle 1 minute, rest 1 minute, cycle 7 minutes, rest 1 minute, cycle 7 minutes, rest 1 minute, cycle 1 minute. Do this 3 times a week.
- *Level 5*—Cycle 1 minute, rest 1 minute, cycle 8 minutes, rest 1 minute, cycle 8 minutes, rest 1 minute, cycle 1 minute. Do this 3 times a week.
- *Level 6*—Cycle 1 minute, rest 1 minute, cycle 9 minutes, rest 1 minute, cycle 9 minutes, rest 1 minute, cycle 1 minute. Do this 3 times a week.
- *Level 7*—Cycle 1 minute, rest 1 minute, cycle 10 minutes, rest 1 minute, cycle 10 minutes, rest 1 minute, cycle 1 minute. Do this 3 times a week.
- *Level 8*—Cycle 1 minute, rest 1 minute, cycle 11 minutes, rest 1 minute, cycle 11 minutes, rest 1 minute, cycle 1 minute. Do this 3 times a week.
- *Level 9*—Cycle 1 minute, rest 1 minute, cycle 12 minutes, rest 1 minute, cycle 12 minutes, rest 1 minute, cycle 1 minute. Do this 3 times a week.
- *Level 10*—Cycle 1 minute, rest 1 minute, cycle 14 minutes, rest 1 minute, cycle 14 minutes, rest 1 minute, cycle 1 minute. Do this 3 times a week.
- *Level 11*—Cycle 1 minute, rest 1 minute, cycle 16 minutes, rest 1 minute, cycle 16 minutes, rest 1 minute, cycle 1 minute. Do this 3 times a week.
- *Level 12*—Cycle 1 minute, rest 1 minute, cycle 18 minutes, rest 1 minute, cycle 18 minutes, rest 1 minute, cycle 1 minute. Do this 3 times a week.
- *Level 13*—Cycle 1 minute, rest 1 minute, cycle 20 minutes, rest 1 minute, cycle 20 minutes, rest 1 minute, cycle 1 minute. Do this 3 times a week.

OBESITY

Generally, the guidelines established in Chapter 4 can be followed by the obese person. Usually, the obese person will feel more comfortable cycling at a lower pulse rate. At first, the duration of exercise may be difficult, but 30 minutes should be tolerated by the time you are eight weeks into the program.

If you are very obese, the arthritic program described in this chapter is a satisfactory alternative.

The programs in this chapter are only general guidelines. Your present health may require you to modify them. They are intended for people who have significant health problems, yet are able to exercise without any complications. As mentioned before, check with your doctor before you begin. '

8

WHOLE-BODY EXERCISES

WORKING THE UPPER body when riding an exercise bike can be a problem. Most exercise bicycles and/or ergometers do not have handlebars that move and allow you to exercise your upper body. Therefore, other exercises are needed to strengthen and firm this part of your anatomy. One alternative is to do a series of exercises with dumbbells. These exercises may be done during the first five minutes of the cycling cool-down or immediately following the cool-down ride but before the stretches. I personally like to do these exercises while pedaling at a slower rate, that is, during the cycling cool-down. Here are the exercises:

Dumbbell Press
- Sit comfortably on the bicycle. Holding a dumbbell in each hand, bring them to shoulder height with your elbows bent, palms facing forward.
- Extend the right arm upward toward the ceiling.
- Return.
- Repeat with the other hand.

Do three sets of 8–15 repetitions. That is, do 8–15 repetitions, rest for a minute, do 8–15 repetitions, rest for a minute, do 8–15 repetitions, rest for a minute, then move on to the next exercise.

Front Raise
- Sit comfortably on the bicycle. Hold a dumbbell in each hand. Hold them in front of your body, resting on the handlebars.
- Keeping the arms straight, slowly raise your arms in an arch until they are directly over your head. (You may raise the arms simultaneously or one at a time.)
- Return to the starting position.
- Repeat.

Do three sets of 8–15 repetitions.

Lateral Raise
- Sit comfortably on the bicycle, holding a dumbbell in each hand at the sides of your body.
- Keeping your arms straight, slowly and simultaneously raise them to the side. Continue upward until your arms are 6–12 inches higher than your head.
- Return to the starting position.
- Repeat.

Do three sets of eight repetitions.

Dumbbell Curl
- Sit comfortably on your bicycle. Grasp a dumbbell in each hand with an overhand grip and allow your arms to hang from your sides.
- By bending your arms at the elbows, slowly alternate curling the weights upward toward your shoulders.
- Return to the starting position.
- Repeat, using each arm.

Do three sets of 8–15 repetitions.

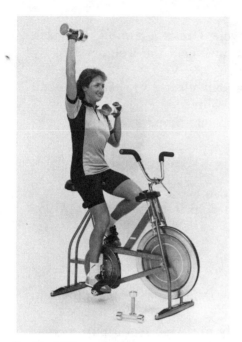

Dumbbell Press

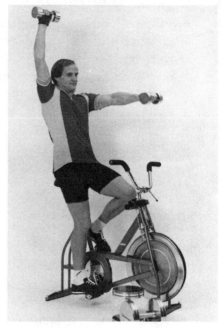

Front Raise

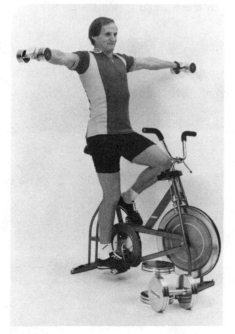

Lateral Raise

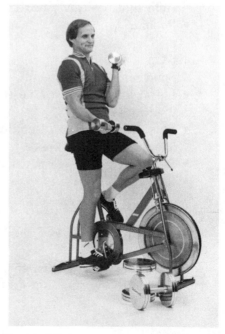

Dumbbell Curl

French Press

- Sit comfortably on your bicycle. Grasp a dumbbell in each hand with an overhand grip and hold the weights directly over your head.
- Slowly and alternately bend your elbows so that your hand (with the weight) drops down behind your back.
- Extend the arm to a full extension above the head.
- Repeat, using each arm.

Do three sets of 8–15 repetitions.

The middle third of your body also needs exercise. Here are a few abdominal exercises that will help to flatten and condition your abdominal muscles:

Curl-Down

Strengthens the abdomen.

- Start from a sitting position on the floor with the knees bent and the hands across the chest.
- Lower the upper body slightly until you feel a pull in your tummy.
- Hold that position and return to the starting position.
- Repeat.

Look-Up

Strengthens the abdomen.

- Lie on your back with the knees slightly bent and the hands on the thighs.
- Raise your head and shoulders from the floor and slide your hands toward the knees.
- Return to the prone position.
- Repeat.

Curl-Up

- Lie on your back with the knees bent and hands/arms across your chest.
- Gradually curl up to a 45-degree angle and hold.
- Return to the starting position.
- Repeat.

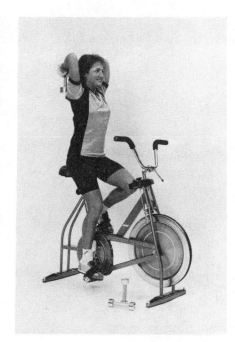

French Press

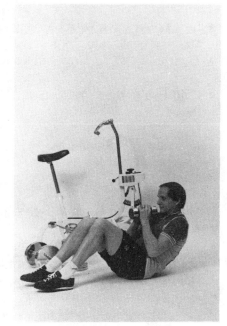

Curl-Down

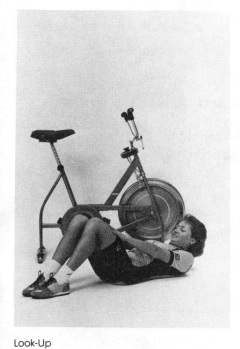

Look-Up

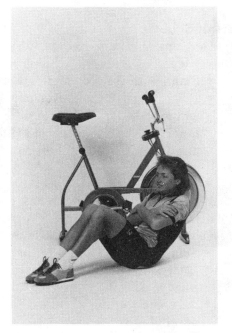

Curl-Up

Pelvic Tilt
- Lie on your back with both legs bent, the feet flat on the floor, and hands at your sides.
- Tighten the abdominal muscles and push the lower back into the floor.
- Hold two to three seconds.
- Repeat.

Your lower body may also need some strengthening. Here are three supplemental leg exercises:

Calf Raise
Develops and firms the muscles in the front and the back of the lower legs.
- Stand with the balls of the feet on a one- to two-inch block of wood or weight plate, heels on the floor.
- Hold a barbell in an overhand grip behind the neck, resting on the shoulders.
- Raise up on the toes as far as possible. Return to the original position. That is one repetition.
- Repeat.

Half Squat
Develops and firms the muscles in the front of the thighs and lower legs.
- Stand with the feet comfortably spread.
- Hold a barbell in an overhand grip behind the neck, resting on the shoulders.
- Bend the knees to perform a Half-Squat (thighs no more than parallel to the floor). Return to the starting position. That is one repetition.
- Repeat

Walking Squat
Develops and firms the muscles of the upper and lower legs.
- Stand with one foot 12–18 inches in front of the other and hold a barbell in an overhand grip behind the neck, resting on the shoulders.
- Take one step forward, executing a Half-Knee-Bend (thighs parallel to the floor).
- Return to the upright position. That is one repetition.
- Repeat the exercise with the other leg.

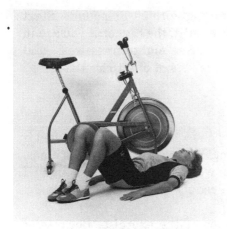

Pelvic Tilt

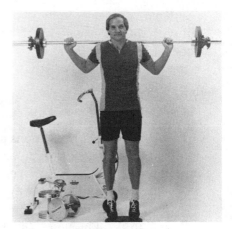

Calf Raise

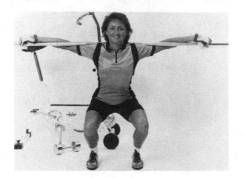

Half Squat

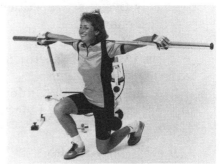

Walking Squat

EXERCISING FOR MUSCLE STRENGTH AND BULK

SCHEDULE

Three exercise sessions a week with at least one day of rest between sessions. All exercises selected (minimum of four) are to be done at each session.

OVERLOAD

Training weights are 50–80 percent of your maximum for the entire exercise. Therefore, if you tested out at 100 pounds for a particular exercise, you will be training with 50–80 pounds. Start out with the lower weights if you are unfit, the higher if you are in good physical condition. Do the exercise eight times, rest, and repeat two more times—that is, three sets of eight repetitions.

PROGRAM

1. Perform eight repetitions of each exercise at a rate you feel is comfortable. Speed is not important. Your goal is eight repetitions, maximum. If you can do more, the weight is not heavy enough. If you cannot do eight, you'll have to reduce the weight.

2. Rest one minute.

3. Attempt eight more repetitions of the exercise. Because of fatigue from the previous eight repetitions, you'll probably be able to do only five or six repetitions.

4. Rest one minute.

5. Repeat the exercise. Again, because of fatigue from the previous two sets of repetitions, you'll probably be able to do only three to five repetitions.

6. After a rest of 1½–2 minutes, proceed to the next exercise in your program, following the same procedure for each exercise.

ADAPTATION AND PROGRESSION

In one to three weeks, your body will adapt to the overload of weight and repetitions. When you can do eight repetitions in each of the three sets for *any* given exercise, add 2½–5 pounds to the barbell or dumbbell. Repeat the cycle of attempting three sets of repetitions for each exercise. After several weeks, when you are able to do three sets of eight, increase the weight by 2½–5 pounds. After several months of training, the increments of increase may be only one to two pounds.

EXERCISE BICYCLES THAT WORK ON THE UPPER BODY

You may be one of the few owners of an exercise bicycle (ergometers that allow you to work on the upper body). These products, while limited in scope, do allow some activation of the upper body when cycling. They may be used by exercisers who have limited leg usage or want a diversion from all-leg training. The arm

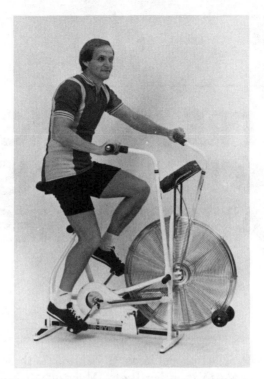

The Schwinn Air-Dyne gives both the arms and legs
a good workout.

movement is rhythmical and, if sustained, has been shown to be
effective in improving cardiovascular fitness—just like leg exercise. But if you want to tone and firm your upper body—arms,
shoulders, back, and chest—stick with the free-weight exercises
recommended at the start of this chapter.

9

PREVENTING ACHES, PAINS, AND OUCHES

THERE ARE SO few problems associated with indoor cycling that I almost hate to mention them. Most of the injuries that do occur do so because too much is done too soon. You cycle too fast, too long, and with too much resistance. As a result, you experience leg, buttocks, arm, and hand pain. If you ride with low-slung handlebars, you may also experience low-back or neck pain.

Most of the following problems can be solved with common sense. If you feel unnatural on the bike or ergometer, try tinkering with it so that it seems to "fit" your body better. If you have pain, the cause is usually twofold: (1) improper fit and (2) too much exercise too soon.

ARM AND HAND COMPLAINTS

Since you grip the handlebars with your hands, this part of your anatomy may experience some problems. If you grip the handlebars too tightly (stressfully), calluses may appear on the palms of the hands. To prevent this problem, do not grasp the bars so tightly, keep changing your hand position as you ride, use foam-rubber-upholstered grips (for a few dollars extra, these can be added), and/or wear padded cycling gloves (see photo).

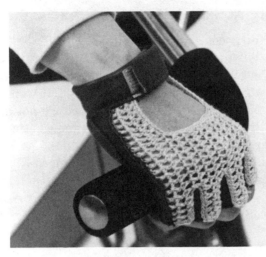

Padded cycling gloves

Since you are exercising indoors, you will not experience the jarring and trauma to the wrist and forearm that an outdoor cyclist does. Therefore, forearm and elbow pains are rare. It is true, however, that some indoor cyclists report tremor or sore muscles in the hands and forearms after unusually long rides. That is particularly true if you have just begun cycling and have a weak upper body or use improper riding techniques.

If you experience this tremor and tingling when first starting your bike fitness program, you'll find that both seem to disappear as your body adapts to the new form of exercise. Conversely, if you really get gung ho on this activity and get carried away, you may find that, after several weeks of training, tingling and tremor appear.

On rare occasions, some cyclists say they experience a numbness or tingling of the fourth and fifth fingers after exceptionally long rides, day after day. Again, this seems to happen mostly with outdoor cyclists, but indoor exercisers have also complained about it. Usually cyclists who use dropped-down handlebars, hold the handlebars too tightly, or have weak, unconditioned upper bodies experience the most problems. The best way to prevent the tingling, numbness, or tremor is to avoid gripping the handgrips tightly, change your hand position frequently when cycling, and make sure you have a proper bike fit (Chapter 3). Upper-body conditioning exercises (Chapter 8) may also help.

SADDLE ACHES, BLISTERS, AND SORES

Saddle aches are fairly common among indoor cyclists. Most of the aches are minor, but they can be aggravating and can keep you from mounting the bike for your "daily constitutional."

Both men and women experience these aches, but women seem to have more problems. Let's face it, bike seats are not designed with the woman in mind (see photo). If I didn't know better, I'd call seat manufacturers sexists. Fortunately, some manufacturers are now enlightened and are offering saddles for women. Women may need to purchase a seat for an outdoor bike, but that's OK; the seat can be fitted nicely on an indoor bike. The Avocet and Brooks B-72 have been designed to accommodate the woman's larger pelvic structure.

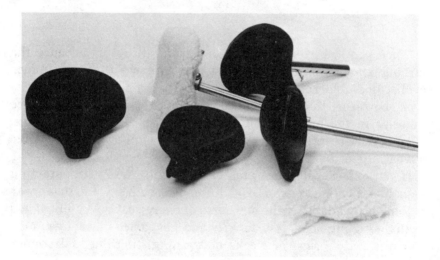

A large variety of bike seats and padding is available.

Some saddle problems include saddle soreness and numb crotch. These are catchall phrases that I think are self-explanatory.

Saddle sores are rare in indoor cycling. A saddle sore is an irritation (hot spot, rash, or breaking of skin) over the ischial tuberositite (the bones you feel right at the bottom of your buttocks). Saddle sores or saddle soreness is usually caused by an improper saddle height. If the saddle is too high or too low, you will slide from side to side. Adjust the seat as described in Chapter 3. Sometimes saddle sores are caused by your pants, shorts, or underwear. The seams and your movement in the saddle can cause irritation, which in time produces blisters or actual saddle sores.

A padded seat may help, as might a new seat. If you're going to sit on a bike or an ergometer for 30 minutes and exercise vigorously, it pays to have a seat designed for your seat.

The tilt of the saddle is also important. If it tilts too far back (or forward), you may experience pressure in your perineum. So make sure the saddle tilt is correct. A proper saddle tilt may reduce the chances of your developing numb crotch. Adjust the saddle as outlined in Chapter 3.

KNEE ACHES

Some indoor cyclists complain of discomfort in the knee. Usually, this is due not to the pedal revolution per minute but to cycling at too high a resistance. That is especially true in the early days of training. People tend to push themselves. Consequently, their muscles, tendons, and ligaments rebel.

Another potential cause of knee problems is the placement of the foot. William Farrell, director of the New England Cycling Academy, states that "the ball of the foot should be positioned over the pedal spindle . . ." Also, if the seat is too high, the tendons and ligaments surrounding the knee are stretched unnaturally. The result is knee pain.

The solutions to knee pain, therefore, include proper pedaling resistance, seat height, and foot placement on the pedal.

NECK AND BACK PAIN

Most neck and back pain occurs during the early days of training. Ways to alleviate the pain depend upon the area of the body.

NECK PAIN

To reduce neck pain, cycle with the head down and your eyes looking upward. Also raise your handlebars or use upright bars. Changing your position frequently will also help. The stretching exercises described in Chapter 4 are helpful as well. Do these *before* and after your ride.

BACK PAIN

To reduce back pain, try one or several of the following:

- Do stretching exercises before and after you ride.
- Move your saddle forward slightly. You'll need to experiment, so move it forward gradually.
- If the saddle is moved forward, raise the saddle and tilt it backward a bit.
- Check the stem of the saddle. It may be too long.
- Change your position as frequently as possible. That is, grip your handlebars at various sites.
- Condition your abdominal muscles with exercises such as Curl-Downs and Look-Ups.
- Last, but not least, give yourself time in the saddle. It may just take you some time to get used to your new activity.

As I said, there are very few aches and pains associated with indoor cycling. Use common sense in your training regimen and make sure your bike and you are a good fit.

10

ACCESSORIES FOR YOUR EXERCISE BIKE

THERE ARE MANY high-tech products available that you can use to measure your heart rate, blood pressure, and calorie expenditure. While some of the more sophisticated ergometers have these devices built in, the average person with a $250 bike does not have that luxury.

To be honest, you don't need these accessories. A watch or clock with a sweep second hand is all you need. With the clock or watch and the ability to take your pulse rate, you can design an excellent exercise program for the indoor bicycle (Chapter 4).

PULSE-RATE DEVICES

There are, of course, some people who have a hard time counting pulse rates, and others don't want (or like) to count their pulses during exercise. Still others do not trust their ability to count the pulse rate. If you are one of the above, you may be interested in one of the pulse rate or heart rate computers, which range in price from $60 to well over $200.

Some of the heart-rate devices are attached to your finger. Some are fastened to your earlobe, and some go around your chest with a belt.

The next question is: Are they accurate? I think a personal illustration is best. I have found that my pulse rate varies greatly when measured by these products. They work well if I stay reasonably still, but when I move, the readings are bizarre. My personal observation plus reactions from many people in my fitness programs have been substantiated by *Bicycling Magazine*. The editors found that the models they tested compared favorably with the local hospital's EKG unit, provided that the user stayed reasonably still. They also found that, when the person moved around on a stationary bicycle seat or moved the finger, some meters gave readings that fluctuated as much as 60 beats. My experience supports their observations.

The units least affected are the ear clip and chest strap. The finger devices proved to be the least reliable.

Genesis Exercise Computer 100 (Biometric Systems, 4040 Del Ray Ave., Marina Del Ray, CA 90291. This computer looks like a huge electronic wristwatch. It weighs about three ounces and has a plastic housing measuring 3 by 2¼ by ⅝ inches. The face is a digital, liquid crystal readout, with three touch controls and a knob for adjusting a metronome. Your pulse rate is picked up by a small band worn near the little finger or another finger. The band connects to the housing on your wrist with a 7-inch wire. Two 1.5-volt batteries provide power.

The Genesis doesn't just record your pulse rate. You can set a pulse rate range, and a beeper will tell you when your rate is above or below these limits. The Genesis will also tell you how long you've kept your rate within these limits and how long it takes your pulse to settle down to a base rate that you set.

There is also a built-in metronome that beeps between 60 and 120 beats per minute, depending upon your wishes (see photo).

Pulse Watch, Model S33-160 (Edmund Scientific Company, 101 E. Glouster Pike, Barrington, NJ 08007, $59.95). This is a watch that has the usual features of a calendar, alarm, and chronograph stopwatch. It also has a built-in monitor on its face. To get a readout, you put your finger on the sensor and wait until the readout stops counting.

Pulse Tach Fingertip Heart Computer (Bay Star, 100 Painters Mill Rd., Dept. 97, Owings Mills, MD 21117). Pulse Tach weighs

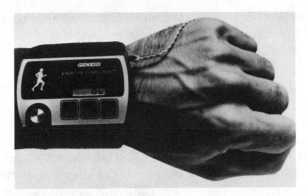

The Genesis Exercise Computer

about 3¾ ounces and is two inches long and an inch wide. It is a miniaturized, digital heart rate meter that fits entirely on the end of your finger. A built-in beeper lets you hear your pulse. There is a one-hour stopwatch to time your recovery and a large liquid crystal, digital display.

The Pulse Tach has an automatic shutoff, long-lasting batteries, and a lanyard to hang around your neck (see photo below).

Amerec 130 (Amerec Corporation, PO Box 3825, Bellevue, WA 98009, $125). This is a simple handlebar monitor for cyclists. The Amerec 130 uses an ear sensor and measures both heart rate and elapsed time. The mounting bracket fits onto the handlebars of your bicycle. A liquid crystal display readout gives you pulse rate and stopwatch simultaneously. Four AAA batteries are included. It measures 4½ by 1 by 3 inches and weighs 6½ ounces.

Amerec 150 Sport Tester Telemeter (Amerec Corporation, PO Box 3825, Bellevue, WA 98009). The Amerec 150 Sport Tester

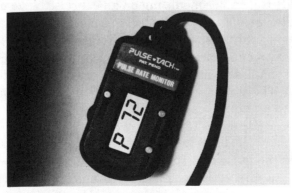

The Bay Star Pulse Tach

Telemeter uses a telemetry system that remotely transmits and receives your heart rate data while you work out.

The Sport Tester Telemeter combines an adjustable chest harness and heart rate transmitter with a receiver that can be hand-held, attached to the wrist, or slipped into the harness holder. This is a short-range telemetry only, about three feet.

The Sport Tester, in addition to monitoring heart rate, can be used as a multifunction programmable training aid. It helps you make the most of your workout by letting you set upper and lower limit alarms at the desired heart rates to keep you working within your training zone. The Amerec 150 also functions as a stopwatch and a clock with a programmable alarm feature. The field transmitter weighs only 1½ ounces, and the microcomputer receiver weighs only 1 ounce.

TE 2000 Sports Tester (distributed by AMF American Inc., 200 American Ave., Jefferson, IA 50129; $250; made in Finland). TE Sports Tester is like the Amerec 150. It uses radio technology to beam your pulse to a small wristwatch monitor. The monitor picks up the signal from a rubber chest strap that contains electrodes similar to those used with EKG machines. There are no wires. The Sport Tester provides information on regular time, elapsed time, and average pulse as well as moment-to-moment readout on where the heart is headed.

1-2-3 Heart Rate Monitor (Country Technology, Inc., PO Box 85, Gays Mills, WI 54631; $295). The 1-2-3 Heart Rate Monitor is a new heart rate meter that supposedly delivers quick, accurate readings without a confusing display of false readings. The first reading (after three rhythmic heart signals) is supposed to be accurate. It is ideal for mounting on an exercise bicycle. The heart rate monitor uses a new ECG electro-sensor that seems to handle perspiration, body oils, and motion. To use the device, you do not need to wear a chest strap harness. You simply place one finger of each hand on the sensors. A four-beat average heart rate is quickly displayed. There is an automatic turnoff and a liquid crystal display (see photo).

Activmeter (Country Technology, Inc., PO Box 87, Gays Mills, WI 54631; $90). The Activmeter is worn on the wrist like a watch and senses the pulse rate with a photo-optic finger sensor. Upper and lower limits activate a warning tone to keep the level of exercise in the proper training range. Heart rate measures are

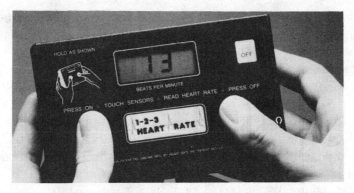

The 1-2-3 Heart Rate Monitor

updated every seven to eight seconds. A time function is also incorporated to time either exercise duration or cardiac recovery time (see photo).

Exersentry Heart Rate Monitor (Respironics, Inc., 650 Seco Rd., Monroeville, PA 15146; $185, plus $17.50 for the bike mounting and $15.00 for the 36-inch cable). The Exersentry uses conductive rubber-sensing electrodes that require no gels. The electrodes fasten to a chest belt and rely on the skin's moisture to sense the heart's electrical system. The Exersentry has a "beeper" with upper and lower alarm limits. You can exercise within your training zone. The Exersentry remains quiet as long as the heart rate remains within the training zone. A miniature earphone is also available to prevent surrounding noise interference. The heart rate display range goes from 40 to over 200 beats per minute. The device weighs three ounces, the electrode belt 6½

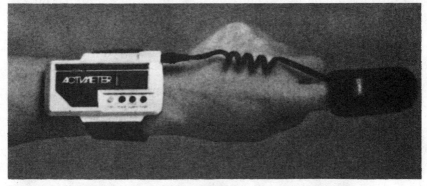

The Activmeter, by Country Technology, Inc.

ounces. The device measures 4 by 2.5 by 1 inch. It requires one 1.5-volt, AAA alkaline battery. A bike-mounting device is also available, along with a 36-inch-long electrode extension cable.

Pulse Meter, Model 110 (Amerec Corporation, PO Box 3825, Bellevue, WA 98009; $139). The Pulse Meter can be mounted on the handlebars of an exercise bicycle. It uses a clothespin-type sensor that you attach to your earlobe. The meter displays your heartbeat in digits and with a light that blinks with each pulse. It can also double as a stopwatch and hour/minute/second mode.

Amerec 160 Vital Signs Monitor (Amerec Corporation, PO Box 3825, Bellevue, WA 98009; $295). The Amerec 160 Vital Signs Monitor provides a printed record of systolic and diastolic blood pressures, heart rate, and body temperature along with the date and time of the readings.

The Amerec 160 has a built-in programmable reminder signal that can be set to alert you to take your measurements at a particular time of the day.

Blood pressure and pulse are taken using the traditional inflation cuff and squeeze bulb, only the function is automatic. Body temperature is measured by a thermal probe, under either the tongue or the armpit.

The compact and lightweight monitor can be powered by batteries for maximum flexibility.

Coach Model S33-106 (Biotechnology, Inc., 6924 NW 46th St., Miami, FL 33166; $199.95). The Coach uses a chest strap with electrodes, with a wire that runs from the strap to a minicomputer. The minicomputer clips onto your waistband. One is available for putting on the front of the bike. The readout runs along the top of the monitor. When you wear it while running, you can measure your distance, calories burned, number of strides, average speed, and elapsed time. When you wear the chest strap, it measures your heart rate and will beep when you exceed your present target pulse rate. You can program it to your needs by punching in data on your sex, age, weight, and resting and target maximum heart rates (see photo).

For $35, the Coach can be adapted for your stationary bike. It is then called the VeloCoach. You program in the wheel circumference so it, too, provides estimates of speed, distance, calories burned, and oxygen uptake.

Caltrac Personal Activity Computer (Hemokinetics, Inc., 2070 Change Bridge Rd., Suite 430, Vienna, VA 22180; $79.95). The

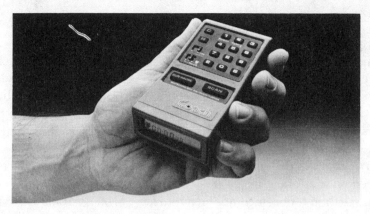

The Coach, by Biotechnology

Caltrac automatically tracks the calories expended. Caltrac's kinetically sensitive computer constantly monitors and logs activity—whether it's walking, standing, or riding a bicycle. All activity is automatically converted into calories expended. Because different bodies burn calories at different rates, Caltrac is programmed to your individual body statistics and calorie intake. Once the proper information is entered, the Caltrac's microcomputer informs you of the calories used. The push of another button provides information regarding calories expended.

CYCLOMETERS

Cyclometers are cyclocomputers that mount on the bike's handlebars and provide a readout on your current speed and mileage, record maximum speed, and then compute average speed. A cyclometer's main purpose is to keep your speed and mileage honest. Several models are available:

- The Avocet Cyclometer 20 sells for $25 and is available from Avocet, PO Box 7615, Menlo Park, CA 94026.
- The Cateye Solar Cyclocomputer sells for $76 and is available from Palo Alto Bicycles, 171 University Ave., Palo Alto, CA 94301. The Cateye has a beeping pacer, a built-in solar cell that eliminates the need for batteries, and an instruction book that is bound to blow you away—four languages.
- The Pacer 2000 ($85) and 2000H ($125) are available from Veltech Sports, 4700 Read St., Boulder, CO 80301.

CHRONOGRAPHS: THE EXERCISER'S WATCH

Chronographs are the watches of the '80s, and they are big business because most people who are into exercise are avid chronograph users. Chronographs are perfect for anyone who is exercising. You can use one to determine your performance based on time. The chronograph is a stopwatch you can carry on your wrist, but it also provides many other features such as pacing, time, alarm, and so forth. In January 1984 the editors of *Runner's World* evaluated the available chronographs. The chart is reproduced on the following page.

More than a dozen companies market chronographs. But virtually all the circuits come from Switzerland and Japan. According to the *Runner's World* group, the Accusplit 934 Turbo stopwatch is the most sophisticated on the market. It seems to do everything but stand on its own head. Not only does it give you the traditional things such as time of day, alarm, light for night use, day, and time, etc.; it can also provide a count-down and count-up time, calculate the elapsed time for a particular distance without erasing the running time, and project your finish time if you know the total distance you are going to go and the split distance.

VIDEOTAPES

VIDEOCYCLE (1020 Green Valley Rd., NW, Albuquerque, NM 87107; $39.95). Recently, videos specifically for indoor cycling have become available. *VIDEOCYCLE* is a 60-minute videotape that contains three self-paced exercise tours specifically designed for indoor cycling. The first two releases of *VIDEOCYCLE* include tours of Grand Teton National Park and Yellowstone National Park.

Besides the spectacular scenery and music, *VIDEOCYCLE* employs some tactics to make each tour a worthwhile exercise experience. Pulse checks, trail maps, and a tour coach help you monitor your progress. Even an occasional on-screen riding companion comes along to join the viewer. Future releases are to be Yellowstone Tour II, Hawaii, and San Francisco.

**Table 21:
Chronographs**

	Composition	Ease of switching modes	Weight	Readability	Sturdiness	Comfort	Overall Rating	Price
Accusplit 930XP	P	8.3	8	9.3	8.3	9	8.5	$39.95
Accusplit 943Turbo	P	8.5	7.5	9.5	8.5	8	8.4	$89.95
Accusplit 932XP	P	8.5	7.5	9.5	8.5	8	8.4	$49.95
RDA Runmaster	P	8.4	7.4	9.5	7.3	7.2	5.9	$79.95
Accusplit 920L	P	6	8.5	6.5	8	9	7.6	$29.95
Seiko Training Timer	M	8.2	6.6	7.2	8.4	7.4	7.56	$95.00
Casio J-50	P	5.8	8.5	8	7.5	7.8	7.52	$29.95
Cronus W-Watch	P	8	9	6	7	7.5	7.4	$39.95
Innovative Pulse Watch	P	8	7.3	7	6.8	6.5	7.1	$74.95
Casio J-30	P	7.6	7.6	6.8	6.4	6.6	7	$24.95
Innovative Ladies' Champion	P	5.5	8.6	5.8	6.6	8.2	6.94	$29.95
Innovative Men's Mariner	P	6.6	7	7.7	6.3	7	6.92	$29.95
Pulsar KB003S	P	8	7.3	6.8	6	6	6.84	$49.50
Accusplit 920XP	P	7	8	6	7	6	6.8	$29.95
Timex 67731	P	4.5	8.6	5.6	6.8	8.2	6.74	$27.95
Chronosport Navigator	P	7.8	4.3	8.8	8	4.8	6.74	$135.00

Key: P = Plastic   Scale 1–10: 1 = unacceptable
      M = Metal   10 = acceptable

11

WHERE TO BUY AN EXERCISE BIKE

SEVERAL COMPANIES SUPPLY exercise bikes and cycle er-gometers. The following names and addresses represent a partial list. These companies provide the actual bike or ergometer and associated components—seats, handlebars, pedals, odometers/speedometers, brake shoes, frames, chain guards, and so on.

Allegheny International
  Exercise Company
US 321 Bypass North
Lincolnton, NC 28093

AJAY
1501 E. Wisconsin St.
Delavan, WI 53115

Amerec Corp.
PO Box 3825
Bellevue, WA 98009

AMF-American
200 American Ave.
Jefferson, IA 50129

AMF-Voit, Inc.
PO Box 958
Santa Ana, CA 92702

AMF-Wheel Good
Olney, IL 62450

AMF-Whitely
29 Essex St.
Maywood, NJ 07607

Atlantic Fitness Products
170-A Penrod Ct.
Glen Burnie, MD 21061

Bally Fitness Products Corp.
10 Thomas Rd.
Irvine, CA 92714

Battle Creek Equipment
307 W. Jackson St.
Battle Creek, MI 49016

Excel
9935 Beverly Blvd.
Pico Rivera, CA 90660

Excelsior Fitness Equipment Co.
615 Landwehr Rd.
Northbrook, IL 60062

Fitness Products
PO Box 254
Hillsdale, MI 49242

BodyGuard—J. Oglaend, Inc.
40 Radio Circle
Mt. Kisco, NY 10549-0096

M & R Industries, Inc.
9215 151st Ave., NE
Redmond, WA 98052

MacLevy Products Corp.
42-23 91st Place
Elmhurst, NY 11373

Marcy Fitness Products
1736 Standard Ave.
Glendale, CA 91201

Monark Bicycle, Imported by:
Quinton Instrument Co.
2121 Terry Ave.
Seattle, WA 98121
and
Universal Fitness Products
20 Terminal Dr., S.
Plainview, L.I., NY 11803

Vitamaster Industries
455 Smith St.
Brooklyn, NY 11231

Walton Manufacturing Co.
106 Regal Rd.
Dallas, TX 75247

Warren E. Collins, Inc.
220 Wood Rd.
Braintree, MA 02184

Exercise bikes and cycle ergometers may also be purchased from local sporting goods stores or discount houses and the following chain stores:

Montgomery Ward
Sears Roebuck and Co.
J. C. Penney

K-Mart
Herman's

WIND TRAINERS AND ROLLERS

Available wind trainers and rollers include the following:

WSI Avenir, available from Western States Imports, Department C, 1837 De Haviland Dr., Newberry Park, CA 91320.
Satuae 2000, Specialized Bicycle Imports, Dept. C, 844 Jury Court, San Jose, CA 95112.

Racer Mate III, Racer Mate, Inc., Dept. C, 3016 N.E. Blakely St., Seattle, WA 98105.

Turbo Trainer, Skid Lid Manufacturing, Dept. C, 1560 California St., San Diego, CA 92101.

HP Criterion, Hooker Performance, Dept. C, 1024 W. Brooks Street, Ontario, CA 91716.

Road Simulator, Slocum Products, Dept. C, 5915 Woodman Ave., Van Nuys, CA 91401.

Vetta, Chan Designs, Dept. C, 1334 B Lincoln Blvd., Santa Monica, CA 91401.

Vortex, Eclipse Inc., Dept. C, PO Box 7370, Ann Arbor, MI 48107.

Tacx Speedbreaker,Veltec Sports, Inc., Dept. C, 4700 Pearl St., #1, Boulder, CO 80301.

Prime, Slocum Products, Dept. C, 5915 Woodman Ave., Van Nuys, CA 91401.

McLain Rollers

Windtrainer I, Brian Co., Inc., Dept. C, 711 E. Gage Ave., Los Angeles, CA 90001.

Windtrainer II, Brian Co., Inc., Dept C, 711 E. Gage Ave., Los Angeles, CA 90001.

Al Kreitler, Al Kreitler Custom Rollers, Inc., Dept. C, 5102 E. Bannister Rd., Kansas City, MO 64137.

Indoor Bike Path, Indoor Bike Path, Dept. C, PO Box 2503, Pasco, WA 99301.

Cinelli Rollers, Consorzio Primo, S.R.L., Dept. C, 10250 Bissonet, Ste. 330, Houston, TX 77036.

APPENDIX

Home Gym Fitness
Exercise Bicycle/Cycle Ergometer Workout Record

Day/ Time	Resting Pulse Rate	mph/kpm	Distance	Time	Exercise Pulse Rate	Comments

Appendix (cont.):
Home Gym Fitness
Exercise Bicycle/Cycle Ergometer Workout Record

Day/ Time	Resting Pulse Rate	mph/kpm	Distance	Time	Exercise Pulse Rate	Comments